DEDICATION

In memory of my mom.

ACKNOWLEDGMENTS

I would first like to thank my friends and family for always being there and for supporting me. I would like to say a special thank you to Andrea Hakanson, who helped me along in this process. And finally, I want to say thank you to all of the people who watched my videos and supported my work; I would never have had this opportunity if it weren't for them.

CONTENTS

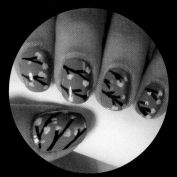

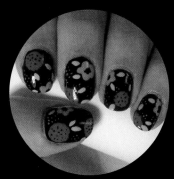

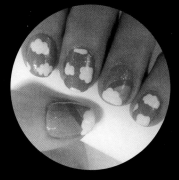

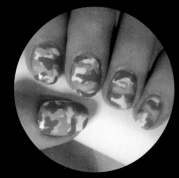

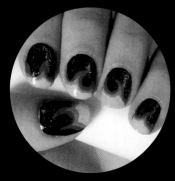

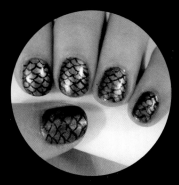

INTRODUCTION

Creating amazing designs is not only fun, but incredibly easy with just a few simple tools. It really requires no experience, and instantly adds a personal shimmer to your nails you can't get anywhere else. You just need to learn a few basic tools and techniques, like which tool is best for making dots, how to create different shapes, and what you'll need to do to your nails to get the best results and achieve the nail art in this book.

The most important thing to remember is this: Practice makes perfect. You shouldn't get discouraged if your first design doesn't come out exactly like the picture. While many of the nail art designs in this book are super easy to recreate, some (like Palm Tree Nails) require a lot of drawing and are hard to get down at first. But don't worry, after a few tries and with the right tools, you'll master these intricate designs and even be able to create your own original ones.

So say goodbye to the nail salon and hello to attention-grabbing nails! With this book, you'll have everything you need to punch up your nails and create fun, one-of-a-kind designs.

HOW TO USE THIS BOOK

You might think that a manicurist or nail technician is the only one who can create beautiful nail designs. After all, they've taken classes and have made a career out of giving thousands of clients the perfect manicure. But designing your nails isn't nearly as scary or difficult as you might think. In fact, once you get started, you'll wonder why you went to the nail salon in the first place. Best of all, you'll have the satisfaction of knowing that you not only accomplished this salon-quality look on your own, but that you didn't have to spend a lot of money doing so. There are just a couple of things you need to know before you get started.

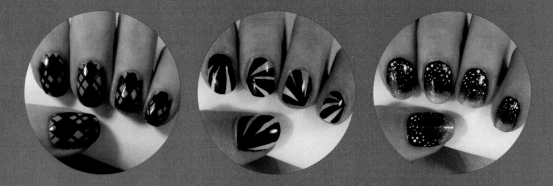

PREPPING YOUR NAILS AND TAKING CARE OF YOUR DESIGN

Creating the perfect manicure and nail art design isn't just about color or pattern. You must allow each nail polish layer to dry as you complete each step in order to make the design last. You also have to make sure that your nails are in good shape. You might be tempted to skip these first few steps, but the prep work is just as essential as the nail art itself. It not only keeps your nails healthy and clean, but extends the polished look of your design. Now, who wouldn't want that?

Cutting and Shaping Your Nails

Before you start any design, you should wipe your nails with a cotton ball soaked in nail polish remover. Even if your nails aren't painted, you should always make this your first step because it helps eliminate any excess oil and allows the nail polish to better adhere to your nail. Then take a nail file or emery board and file your nails into one of the five common nail shapes: oval, square, pointed, squoval, or round. If you've been to a nail salon before, you may already know what shape suits your fingers best, but if not, a simple Google search will give you images and descriptions of these nail shapes. Something you can do to make your nails look longer is push the cuticle back. You'll need to soak your hands in warm water to help soften the cuticle,

then push it back with an orange stick. Finally, trim any hangnails around your nails with a pair of nail clippers. You should also apply a moisturizer after you've completed your design to help keep your nails looking this way.

These simple steps will instantly clean up your nails and give you the foundation you need to successfully create your nail art.

Base Coat and Top Coat

A base and top coat can also add a professional touch to your nail art. A base coat will preserve your natural nail and create a smooth canvas to work on, while the top coat seals in your design.

They are sold under many different brands and range from strengthening to nonstaining types. It's good to use both a base coat and a top coat since they give both your natural nail and your nail art the best possible protection against stains and chips.

After you've prepared your nails, the first nail polish you should paint onto them is the base coat. Base coats fill in lines and cracks on your nails, so your nail color has an even surface to adhere to. This will not only make your manicure last longer, but will also provide a barrier that prevents dark colors from staining your natural nail. While any clear base coat will do the trick, you might want to consider investing in a formula fortified with protein, Vitamin E, and/or calcium, as these elements replenish the nutrients and moisture in your nails and prevent damage like splitting or peeling.

Like the base coat, a top coat polish is a clear protective polish. Applied after your nail art is complete, the top coat seals in your design and prevents the color from fading. It also adds shine to the look, and when it is reapplied during the week, it will help prevent chipping. When applying a top coat, make sure to paint underneath your tips as well, since this makes the manicure last much longer.

TOOLS AND TECHNIQUES

While every piece of nail art is different, there are a few things you should keep on hand when you're creating a design. Your go-to nail art kit should include a dotting tool, a nail art brush, nail decals, a palette, a top coat, and the nail colors you're using. These tools are very inexpensive and can be found in beauty supply stores and online at websites like *www.amazon.com* or *www.ebay.com*. For nail color, any brand will do as long as it's opaque and coats your nail well. The more specialized nail tools, like the nail art brush, make your life easier when you're creating intricate designs. That said, it's easy to be creative and improvise if you don't have a certain specific tool at hand. For every tool that is discussed, this book suggests household items that make great substitutions for creating the same effect. No matter what tool you use, be sure to clean it with nail polish remover after you finish the design in order to extend its life and get a clean look every time.

Dotting Tool

A great first tool for those looking to get into nail art is the dotting tool. This tool is incredibly easy to use. It has a long handle with a small round ball at each tip (some dotting tools will only have one tip). As you can probably guess by the name, dotting tools are primarily used to create dots, but that doesn't mean that your nail art has to be simple or boring. You can use the dotting tool to create flowers, a starry sky, and even enhance designs with a few strategic dots. To use a dotting tool, simply drip some nail polish on a nonporous surface, like a palette or a piece of paper, dip the tool in it, and dot your nail. The key here is to coat the ball at the top of the tool with enough nail color to create the appropriate size of dot—the more you add, the bigger your dot will be. If you need to create small dots but can't find a dotting tool, you can use a toothpick, the end of a sewing pin, or even the rounded end of a bobby pin. For larger dots, the end of a paintbrush or makeup brush handle work well.

Nail Art Brush

The nail art brush is another tool that you'll want to invest in if you're interested in doing more complex designs. There are a variety of styles and sizes on the market, so make sure you consider what type of art you want to create before making a purchase. If you'll still not sure of what kind of brush you'll need, many stores offer a nail art brush kit that comes with a selection of brushes in various shapes and sizes. For the nail art in this book, however, You should use a thin brush with fine bristles. This brush, sometimes called a detailing brush, allows for more intricate designs like leaves or roses. It also makes it easier to draw straight lines, but it will take some time to get used to if you don't have a steady hand. If you have a hard time holding the brush, try rotating the hand you are working on instead of the hand you are painting with. Pivoting the hand you're painting will help you create even lines. To use a detailing brush, place drops of nail polish on a nonporous surface, dip the tip of the brush into the nail polish, and paint a design onto your nails just like you would with a paintbrush. Be careful to never dip the nail art brush into the nail polish bottle, though, as this can lead to unwanted drips and messy designs. If you're looking for a great alternative to using a nail art brush, you can use a small makeup brush, an eyeliner brush, or a small paintbrush instead. If you're using a paintbrush, however, you'll want to trim the bristles down to the appropriate shape and size for your design. You should always make sure to clean your brushes in between steps in order to extend their life and create a clean design. To do this, you can dip the brushes in pure acetone nail polish remover and wipe the tips off with a dry paper towel. If you're using acrylic paint for your nail art designs, you can clean the brushes by simply rinsing the tips in lukewarm water.

Nail Decals

Nail decals are tiny stickers that you can easily apply to your nails using a pair of tweezers. They come in all sorts of designs, such as flowers, stars, hearts, and materials like rhinestones. Several designs come on a single transfer sheet. If you're applying rhinestones, gently press the decal onto your nail before your nail polish dries, then seal it all with a top coat once the polish is dry. For a regular decal, apply it to your nails after your nail polish has dried and apply a top coat over the design. While not all of the nail art designs in this book require nail decals, you can apply a few stickers to your nails to add your own touch and really make your favorite design pop.

Acrylic Paint

Acrylic paint has been used by manicurists and nail technicians for years. Since acrylic paint can be mixed to create a variety of different colors, it is a cheaper alternative to using nail polish and can help you add details without having to own a vast nail polish collection. It is also a great beginner's tool because it can easily be wiped away if a mistake is made before it dries. When using acrylic paint, you should always apply a base coat and a nail color first since the paint should only be used to add details and will not provide the lustrous color of a nail polish.

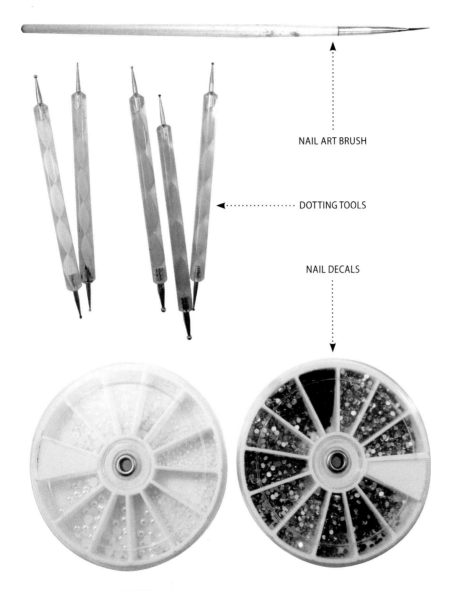

NAIL ART BRUSH

DOTTING TOOLS

NAIL DECALS

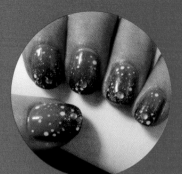

NAIL ART DESIGNS

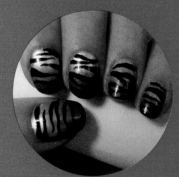

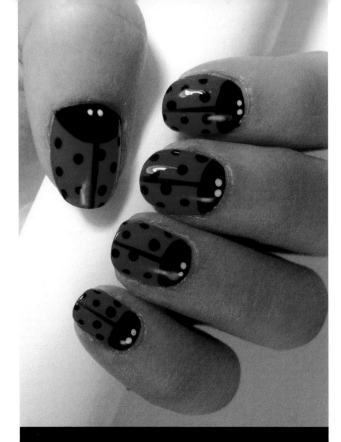

LADYBUG NAILS

These adorable ladybug nails are great for the summertime. They can be worn on all your nails, or on just a couple as a fun accent.

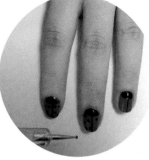

1   Start by painting your nails with a bright red nail polish.

5   Using the larger tip of a dotting tool and a black nail polish, create random dots on either side of the black line you drew down the center of your nail.

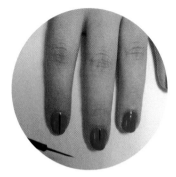

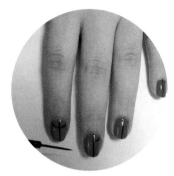

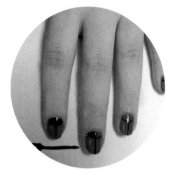

2 Dip a thin nail art brush into a black nail polish and create a straight line right down the center of your nail.

3 Using the same brush and nail color, create a half-circle shape at the base of your nail.

4 Fill in the half circle with black nail polish.

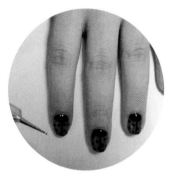

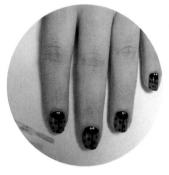

6 Using a smaller end of the dotting tool and white nail polish, create two tiny dots in the black half circle you created. These will be the ladybug's eyes.

7 Finally, apply a top coat to your nails to seal in the design.

VINTAGE ROSE NAILS

A simple floral print nail art design, perfect for spring! This eye-catching design will surely bring a vintage look to any outfit.

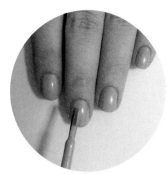

1   Start by painting your nails with a nude beige nail polish.

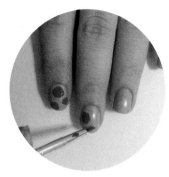

2   Using a small nail art brush, create a few circles on each nail. The circles don't need to be perfect.

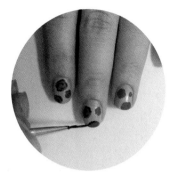

3   Using a thinner brush and a dark red nail polish, carefully outline each rose, then do several smaller C-shapes within the circle to suggest petals.

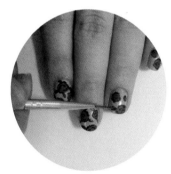

4   Using the same thin brush and a dark green nail polish, lay the brush down on your nail to make oval-shaped leaves around each rose.

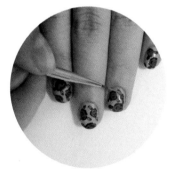

5   Using the same thin brush and a lighter green nail polish, add some details to the leaves.

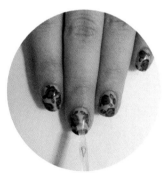

6   Finally, apply a top coat to your nails to seal in the design.

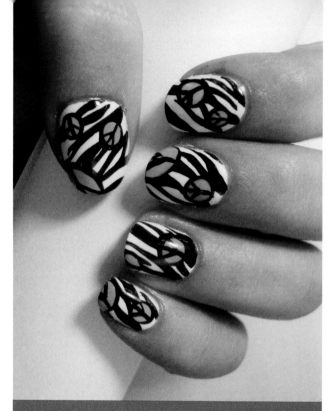

NEON PEACE SIGN ZEBRA NAILS

This is a funky nail design that will brighten your day. If you love animal prints and bright colors, this design has it all.

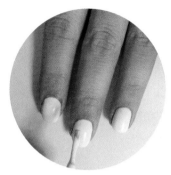

1 Start by painting your nails with a white nail polish.

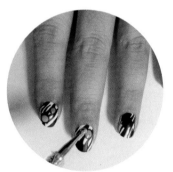

4 Using the dotting tool and neon nail colors, such as pink and green, fill in the black circles with the neon colors.

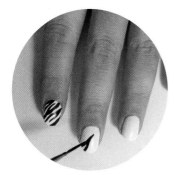

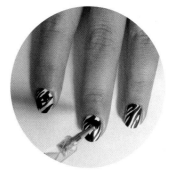

2 Using a thin nail art brush and a black nail polish, create wavy lines on your nails starting at the bottom of your nail and moving up diagonally.

Make sure you create waves going in both directions and fill in any large gaps with more waves.

3 With a dotting tool and the black nail polish, place small and large dots on top of the zebra pattern you just created.

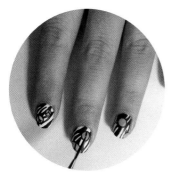

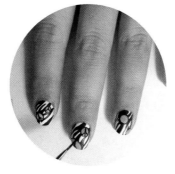

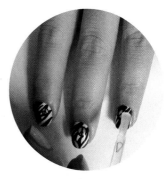

5 With a thin nail art brush and the black nail polish, draw a line straight down the middle of the circle.

6 In order to complete the peace sign, make an inverted V-shape stemming from the center line.

7 Finally, apply a top coat to your nails to seal in the design.

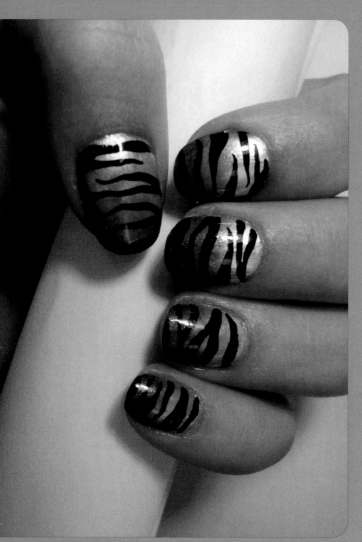

BLUE FADED ZEBRA NAILS

A simple zebra print design with a twist. Create this beautiful faded look with any of your favorite colors.

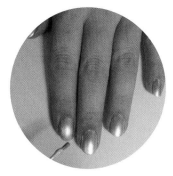

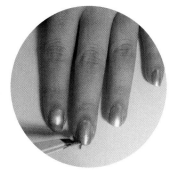

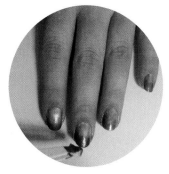

1 Start by painting your nails with a silver nail polish.

2 Using a small piece of a cosmetic sponge and some tweezers, apply a deep blue nail polish to your nails. Leave the top third of your nails mostly silver to create a transitional gradient effect.

3 Dab on a darker blue nail polish using the same method, but this time focus on the tips of your nails.

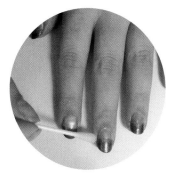

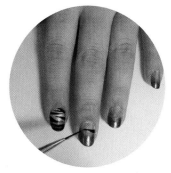

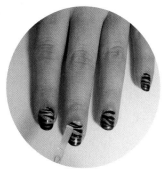

4 Using a Q-tip and acetone, remove any nail polish that landed on your skin.

5 Using a thin nail art brush and a black nail polish, create wavy lines starting at the top of your nail moving down diagonally.

6 Finally, apply a top coat to your nails to seal in the design.

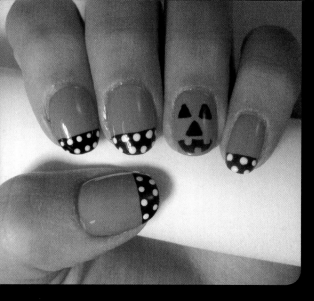

HALLOWEEN JACK-O'-LANTERN NAILS

Celebrate Halloween by dressing up your nails with this haunting design!

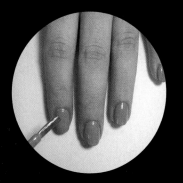

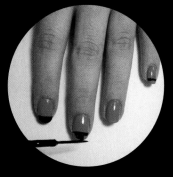

1 Start by painting your nails with a bright orange nail polish.

2 Using a thin nail art brush and a black nail polish, create a straight French tip on all of your nails except the ring finger. You can also freehand it with the nail polish brush if you don't own a nail art brush.

3 Using the same brush and nail color, fill in the French tips.

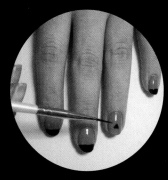

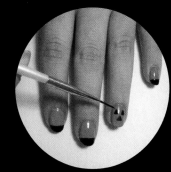

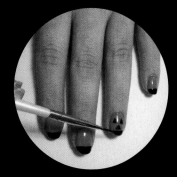

4 Using a thinner nail art brush and the same nail color, draw a simple triangle in the center of your ring finger nail. This will be the jack-o'-lantern's nose.

5 Using the same brush and nail color, draw two triangles, one on each side of the first triangle, to be the jack-o'-lantern's eyes.

6 Using the same brush and nail color, create your jack-o'-lantern's mouth by drawing a half circle at the bottom of your nail.

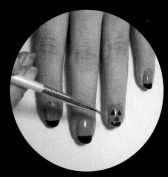

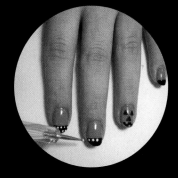

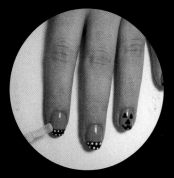

7 Once the half circle is dry, use a nail art brush and the bright orange nail polish to draw a few small squares along the top of the half circle. These squares will be your jack-o'-lantern's teeth.

8 Using a small dotting tool and a white nail polish, create polka dots on your black tips.

9 Finally, apply a top coat to your nails to seal in the design.

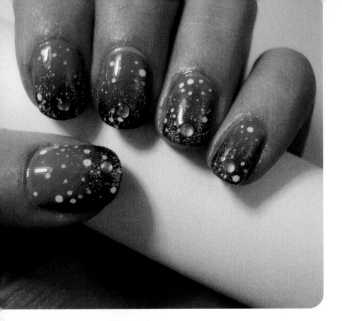

FOREST PIXIE NAILS

A fairytale nail design perfect for anyone who wants to add a little adventure to her wardrobe.

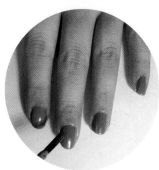

1 Start by painting your nails with a medium green nail polish.

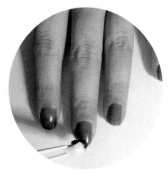

2 Using a small piece of a cosmetic sponge and some tweezers, apply a dark green nail polish to your nails. Leave the top third of your nails mostly medium green.

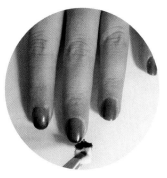

3 Dab on a black nail polish using the same method, but this time focus on the tips of your nails.

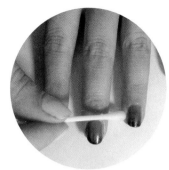

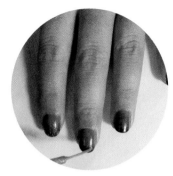

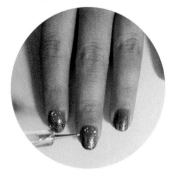

4 Using a Q-tip and acetone, remove any nail polish that landed on your skin.

5 Apply a gold glitter polish over the tips of your nails.

6 Using a dotting tool and a white nail polish, make small dots in various sizes to look like sparkles.

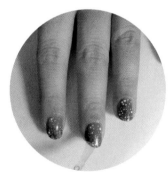

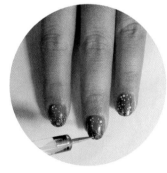

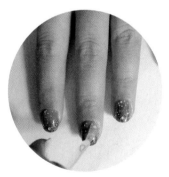

7 Apply a top coat to your nails.

8 Before the top coat dries, carefully place a yellow rhinestone decal on each of your tips with a pair of tweezers or dotting tool.

9 Finally, apply a top coat to your nails to seal in the design.

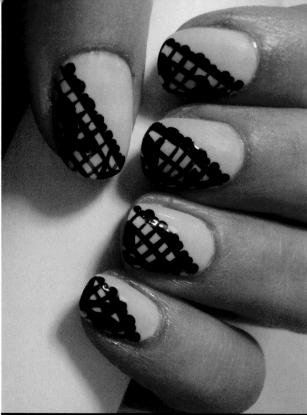

BLACK LACE NAILS

This simple and elegant lace over a nude background gives a feminine look to your manicure.

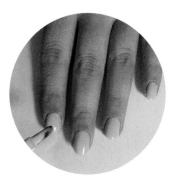

1 Start by painting your nails with a light beige nail polish.

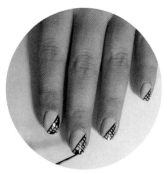

5 Using the same nail art brush and nail polish, draw small leaves and stem shapes inside the crisscross pattern to create a lace effect.

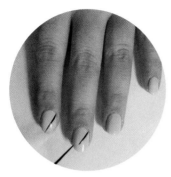

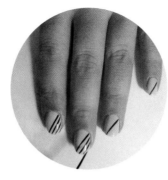

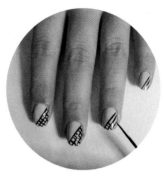

2 Using a thin nail art brush and a black nail polish, create a diagonal line on each of your nails from one corner of the nail to the other.

3 Continue making a row of diagonal lines below the first diagonal line you created with the nail art brush and the black nail polish.

4 Angle your fingers slightly and create another row of lines over the first set of diagonal lines. This will make a crisscross pattern.

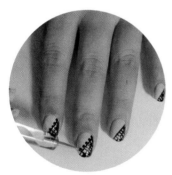

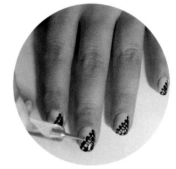

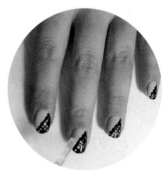

6 Using a dotting tool and the black nail polish, place small dots along your first diagonal line to create a scalloped edge.

7 With the same tool and nail polish, place smaller dots between the previous dots.

8 Finally, apply a top coat to your nails to seal in the design.

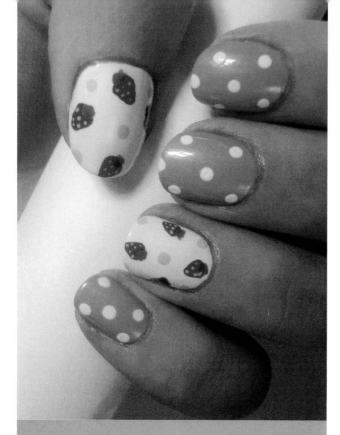

STRAWBERRIES AND POLKA DOT NAILS

This fresh strawberry manicure with cute polka dots will make your fingers look good enough to eat.

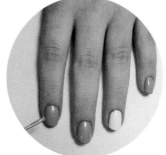

1 Start by painting your ring finger and thumb nails with a white nail polish. Then paint the rest of your nails with a light pink nail polish.

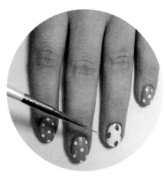

5 Using the same nail art brush and a yellow nail polish, place tiny yellow dots inside the strawberries. These will be the seeds.

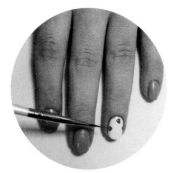

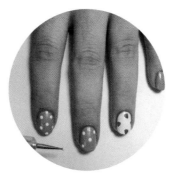

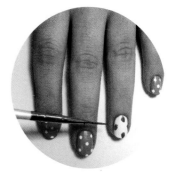

2 Using a thin nail art brush and a red nail polish, begin making small upside down triangular shapes on the white nails. Make sure that the triangles are slightly rounded, since they will be your strawberries.

3 Using a dotting tool and a white nail polish, place dots in a polka dot pattern on all of the pink nails.

4 Using a thin nail art brush and a green nail polish, draw a few leaves above the strawberries.

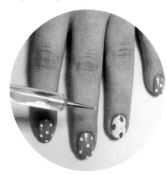

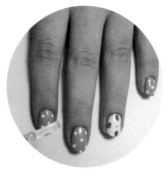

6 Using a dotting tool and the light pink nail polish, fill in the empty area between the strawberries with polka dots.

7 Finally, apply a top coat to your nails to seal in the design.

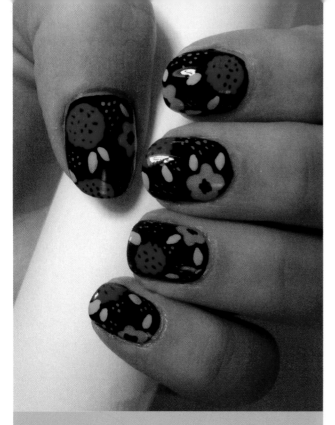

'80s FLORAL NAILS

A gorgeous floral pattern inspired by the retro '80s print. Bright colors layered over a dark background will bring a pop of color to your nails.

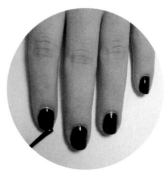

1 Start by painting your nails with a black nail polish.

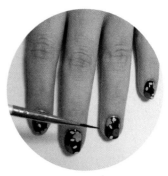

5 Using the nail art brush and a black nail polish, place small dots inside the red flowers.

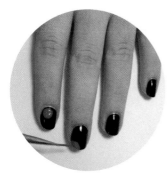

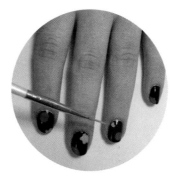

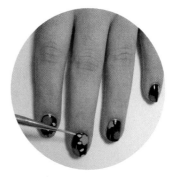

2 Using a small nail art brush and a red nail polish, roughly draw circles on your nails. These will become your retro flowers.

3 Using the same nail art brush and a bright pink nail polish draw additional flower shapes.

4 Using the same tool and a neon green nail polish, add small leaves by laying the brush down close to the flowers.

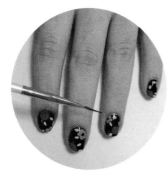

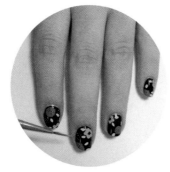

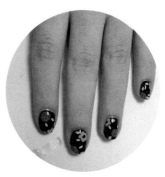

6 Using the same tool and nail polish, fill in the center of the pink flowers with a large black circle.

7 Using a thin nail art brush and a light blue nail polish, draw dots in any empty areas of your nails.

8 Finally, apply a top coat to your nails to seal in the design.

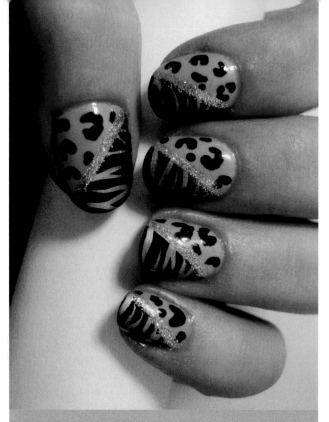

PINK AND BLACK ANIMAL PRINT NAILS

Animal prints are always fun! Mix up the patterns with this cute zebra and leopard print design.

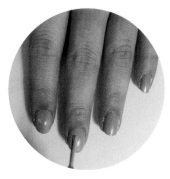

1   Start by painting your nails with a soft pink nail polish.

5   Using the same nail art brush and nail polish, create silver wavy lines horizontally inside the black area. These lines will be the zebra pattern.

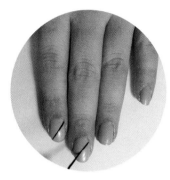

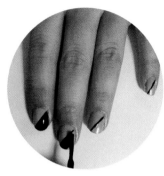

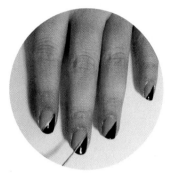

2 Using a thin nail art brush and a black nail polish, draw a diagonal line from one corner of your nail to the other.

3 Fill in the bottom half of the nail with black nail polish.

4 Using the nail art brush and a silver nail polish, draw a diagonal line along the very top of the black section to create a silver border between the pink and black areas.

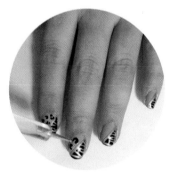

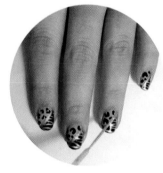

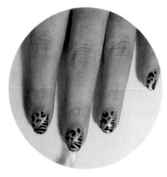

6 Using a small dotting tool and the black nail polish, create C-shapes and spots on the pink half of your nails. These will be the leopard spots.

7 Apply a silver glitter nail polish over the silver line.

8 Finally, apply a top coat to your nails to seal in the design.

SUMMER CITRUS NAILS

Perfect for the hot summer months, this bright citrus design is a refreshing style for your nails.

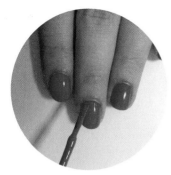

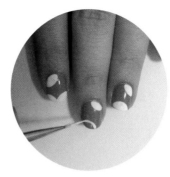

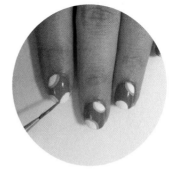

1 Start by painting your nails with a coral nail polish.

2 Using a nail art brush and a white nail polish, create half circles of different sizes along the edges of your nails, and fill them in.

3 With a nail art brush and either a green, orange, or yellow nail polish, outline each of the circles. This outline will be the rind of a citrus slice.

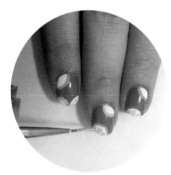

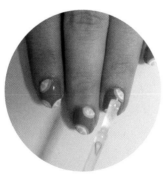

4 Using the same brush and nail colors, create small teardrop shapes inside the circles. These will be the wedges in a citrus slice, so make sure the color of your teardrop shape matches the outline color.

5 Finally, apply a top coat to your nails to seal in the design.

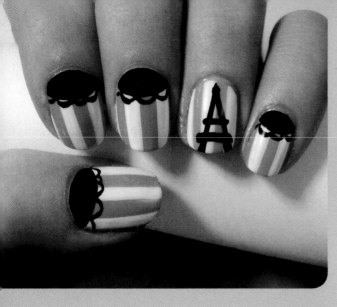

PARIS-INSPIRED NAILS

This nail design will whisk you away to the romantic city of Paris.

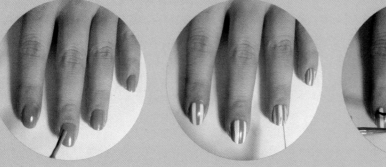

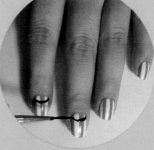

1 Start by painting your nails with a light pink nail polish.

2 Using a nail art brush and a white nail polish, begin making vertical stripes on all of your nails.

3 Using a nail art brush and a black nail polish, draw a half-moon shape at the base of each nail except the ring finger nails.

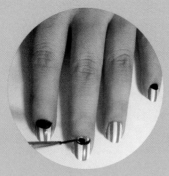

4 Using the same brush and nail polish, fill in the half-moon shapes.

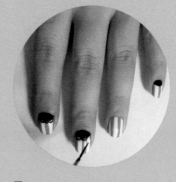

5 Using the tip of the nail art brush, draw black loops along each black half-moon shape to create a lacy scalloped edge.

6 Using the same nail art brush and nail polish, draw a black A-shape on your ring finger nails.

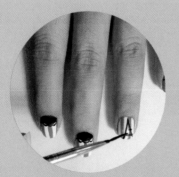

7 Using the same nail art brush and nail polish, draw two horizontal lines inside the A-shape, one at the top and another closer to the bottom, to create the Eiffel Tower.

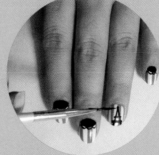

8 Using the same nail art brush and nail polish, place a large black dot at the top of the Eiffel Tower.

9 Finally, apply a top coat to your nails to seal in the design.

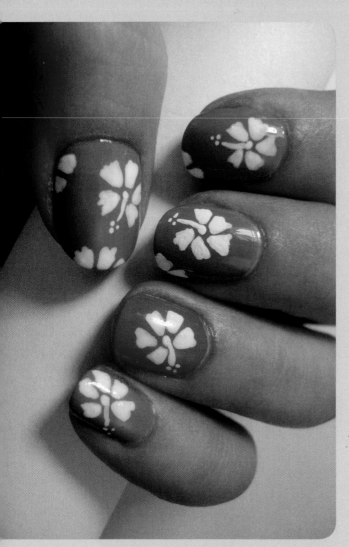

HAWAIIAN HIBISCUS NAILS

This tropical manicure will have you dreaming of the beach!

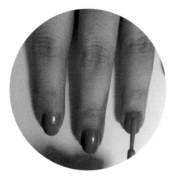

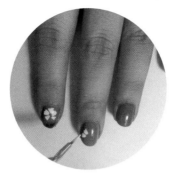

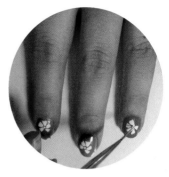

1 Start by painting your ring finger nails with a bright pink nail polish. Paint the rest of your nails with a bright blue nail polish.

2 Using a nail art brush and a white nail polish, draw five triangular-shaped petals stemming from a center point.

3 With the tip of the brush, place a white dot in the center of each flower.

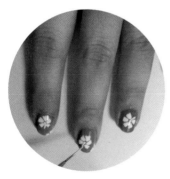

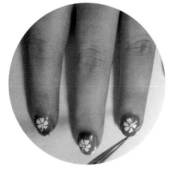

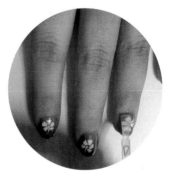

4 Using the same brush and nail polish and starting from the center of the dot, draw a line radiating out of the flower.

5 Using the same tool and nail polish, place three small dots at the end of it. These will be the stamen of the hibiscus.

6 Finally, apply a top coat to your nails to seal in the design.

NAUTICAL NAILS

Make waves and be on trend with these nautical theme nails!

1 Start by painting your nails with a navy blue nail polish.

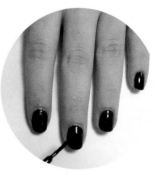

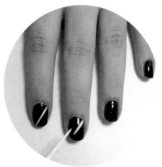

2 Using a nail art brush and a white nail polish, draw a diagonal line from one corner of your nail to the other on all of your nails except the ring finger.

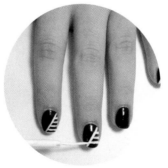

3 Using the same tool and nail polish, create horizontal lines filling in the area inside the bottom half of each nail.

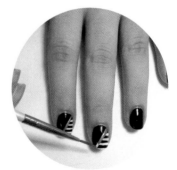

4 Using a nail art brush and a gold nail polish, paint a gold line over the white diagonal across the center of the nail.

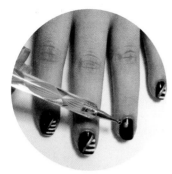

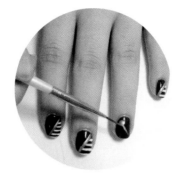

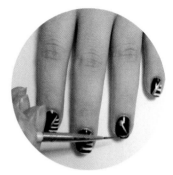

5 Using a dotting tool and the same nail polish, make a large gold dot in the upper corner of each of your ring finger nails.

6 Using a nail art brush and the same nail polish, create a line stemming diagonally from the dot. This will be the shank of the anchor.

7 Using the same tool and nail polish, draw a gold curved line at the end of the shank to create the flukes of the anchor.

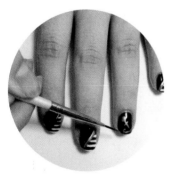

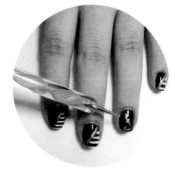

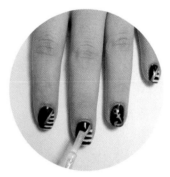

8 Using the same tool and nail polish, draw small gold arrows at the ends of the curved line, and a small horizontal line across the top of the shank line, right underneath the gold dot.

9 Using a dotting tool and the navy blue nail polish, place a dot inside the gold one to create the hole in the top of the anchor.

10 Finally, apply a top coat to your nails to seal in the design.

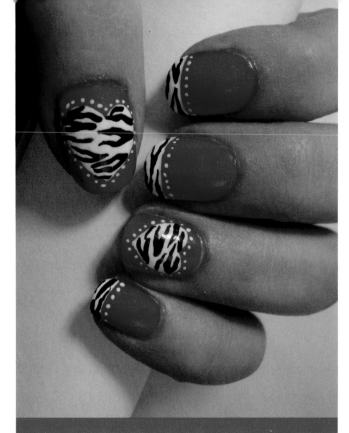

HOT PINK ZEBRA NAILS

An extremely girly nail design, showing a love for zebra print and the color pink.

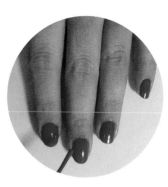

1 Start by painting your nails with a hot pink nail polish.

5 Using a nail art brush and a black nail polish, draw wavy lines horizontally on all the white areas to create a zebra print.

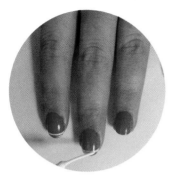

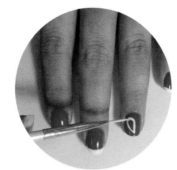

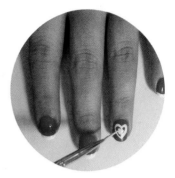

2 Using a thin nail art brush and a white nail polish, create a French tip on all your nails except the ring finger nails.

3 Using the same nail art brush and nail polish, draw a white heart in the middle of each of your ring finger nails.

4 Fill in the hearts with white nail polish.

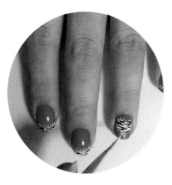

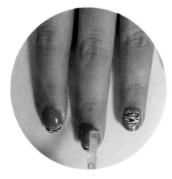

6 Using the same nail art brush and the white nail polish, place small dots along the French tip and around the heart.

7 Finally, apply a top coat to your nails to seal in the design.

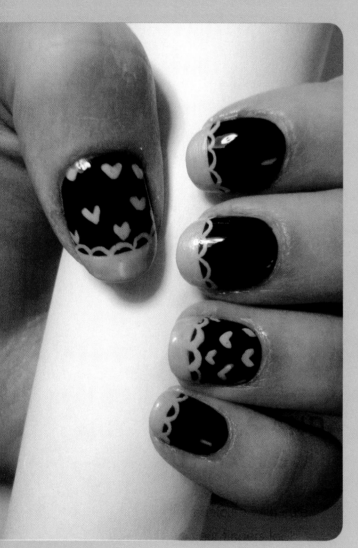

SWEETHEART PINK NAILS

A sweet pink and brown nail design, ideal for Valentine's Day.

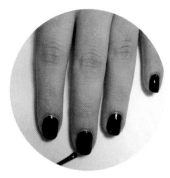

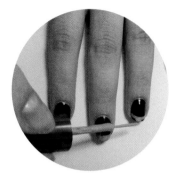

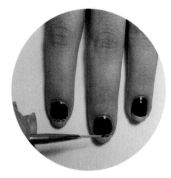

1 Start by painting your nails with a dark chocolate brown nail polish.

2 Using a nail art brush and a pink nail polish, create French tips. You can also freehand it with the nail polish brush.

3 Using the same nail art brush and nail polish, draw loops along the tips to give your nails a lace look.

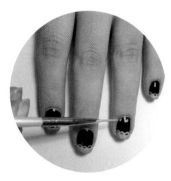

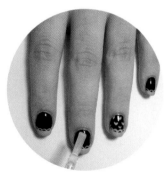

4 Using the same nail art brush and nail polish, create small rounded V-shapes, or hearts, on each nail.

5 Finally, apply a top coat to your nails to seal in the design.

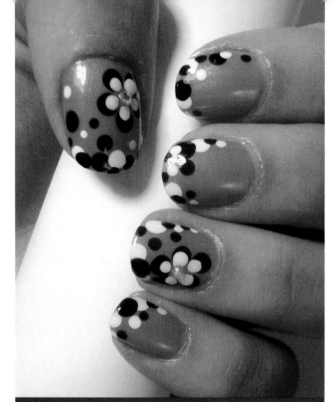

FLOWERS AND BUBBLES NAILS

Perfect for beginners, this simple and quick nail art design will add an elegance to plain nails.

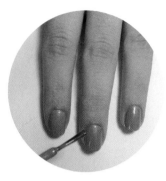

1 Start by painting your nails with a pink nail polish.

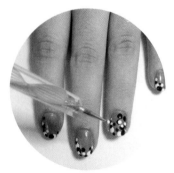

5 Place smaller white dots over the purple ones you've just made, to define the petals.

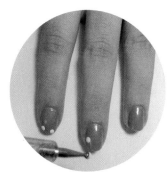

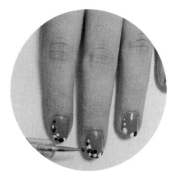

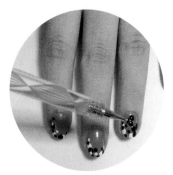

2 Using a dotting tool and a white nail polish, place large and small dots on the tips of your nails.

3 Repeat Step 2 with a dark purple nail polish. It's okay if any of the dots overlap.

4 Using the dotting tool and the purple nail polish, place five large dots in a circular shape to create a flower on your thumb and ring finger nails.

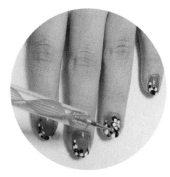

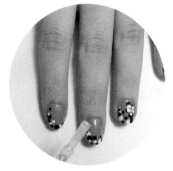

6 Carefully use a pair of tweezers or a dotting tool to place a white decal in the center of the flower.

7 Finally, apply a top coat to your nails to seal in the design.

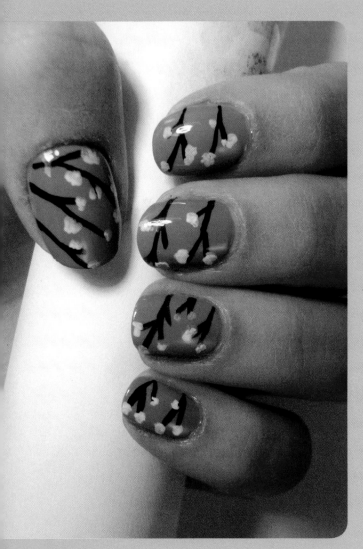

CHERRY BLOSSOM NAILS

A beautiful floral nail design inspired by the blossoms of the cherry tree.

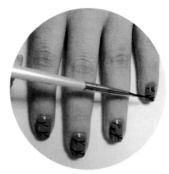

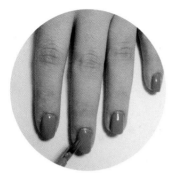

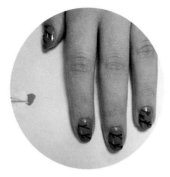

1 Start by painting your nails with a sky blue nail polish.

2 Using a thin nail art brush and a dark brown nail polish, draw the branches of the tree.

3 Mix a pink and a white nail polish together in a palette with a nail art brush or toothpick and dip the tip of your brush into your new color.

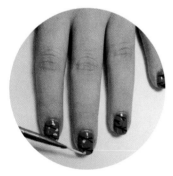

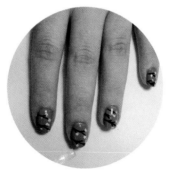

4 Using a thin nail art brush and the light pink you've mixed, place dots of varying sizes all along the branches to make the flowers.

5 Finally, apply a top coat to your nails to seal in the design.

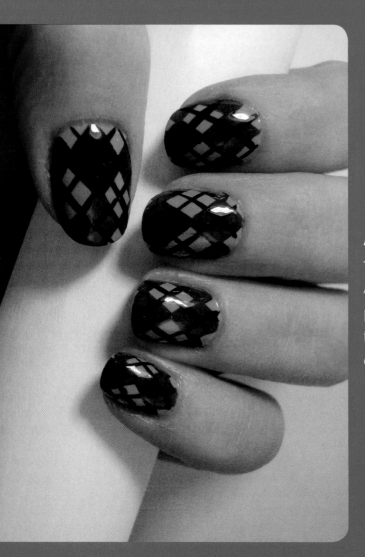

ARGYLE NAILS

A cute and simple argyle pattern. Switch up the colors to match your mood or your outfit!

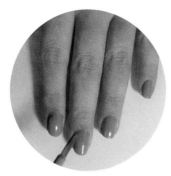

1 Start by painting your nails with a grey nail polish.

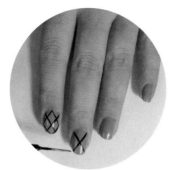

2 Using a thin nail art brush and a black nail polish, create a crisscross pattern on all of your nails.

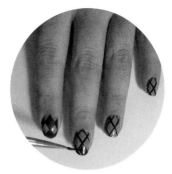

3 Using a thin nail art brush and a dark grey nail polish, fill in every other square.

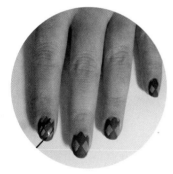

4 Using a thin nail art brush and the black nail polish, create a set of diagonal lines starting from the top right corner of your nails.

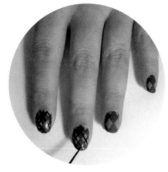

5 Using the same tool and nail polish, create another set of diagonal lines starting from the top left corner of your nails.

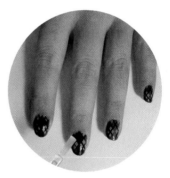

6 Finally, apply a top coat to your nails to seal in the design.

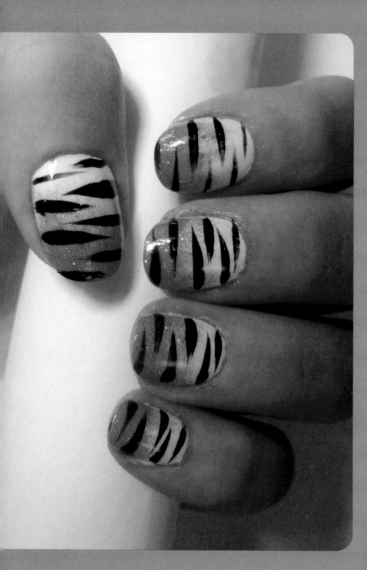

TIGER PRINT NAILS

This fierce tiger print nail art uses a trendy gradient effect to make it pop.

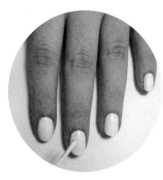

1 Start by painting your nails with a white nail polish.

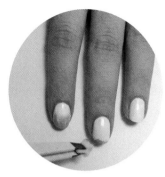

2 Using a small piece of a cosmetic sponge and some tweezers, apply a light orange nail polish to your nails. Leave the top third of your nails mostly white.

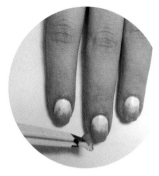

3 Using the same method, dab a dark orange nail polish on the tips of your nails.

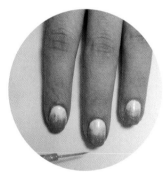

4 Apply a thin layer of gold glitter nail polish over the orange area.

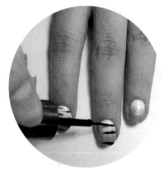

5 Using a thin nail art brush and a black nail polish, draw tiger stripes from each side extending into the center of the nail.

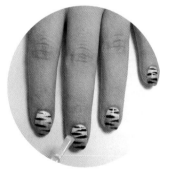

6 Finally, apply a top coat to your nails to seal in the design.

TURQUOISE AND GOLD LEOPARD PRINT NAILS

An edgy, modern twist on the original leopard print colors.

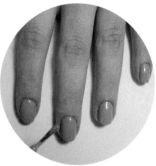

1 Start by painting your nails with a turquoise blue nail polish.

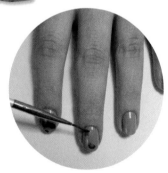

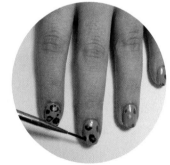

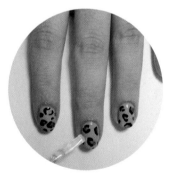

2 Using a nail art brush and a gold nail polish, place random dots on your nails. Don't worry about the dots being perfectly round; a leopard's spots are slightly irregular.

3 Using a nail art brush and a black nail polish, draw C-shapes around the edges of the dots.

4 Finally, apply a top coat to your nails to seal in the design.

DAISY NAILS

These bright floral daisy nails are great for springtime!

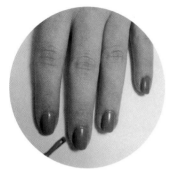

1 Start by painting your nails with a green nail polish.

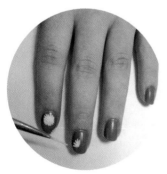

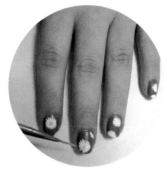

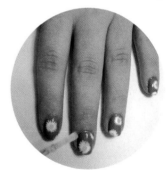

2 Using a nail art brush and a white nail polish, outline a circle on your nail. Draw straight lines radiating out from the circle to make petals.

3 Using a nail art brush and a yellow nail polish, place a cluster of yellow dots in the center of the circle.

4 Finally, apply a top coat to your nails to seal in the design.

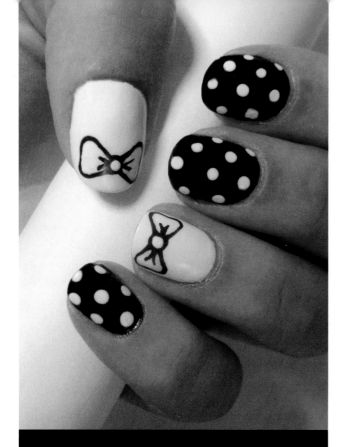

CUTE BOW NAILS

This chic polka dot design adds a touch of cuteness with an accent bow.

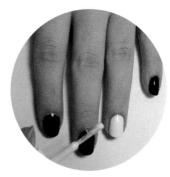

1   Start by painting your ring finger and thumb nails with a white nail polish. Paint the rest of your nails with a black nail polish.

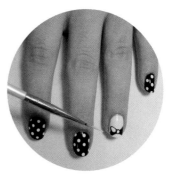

5   Using a nail art brush and the white nail polish, fill in the heart shapes and black dot, but leave a thin black outline.

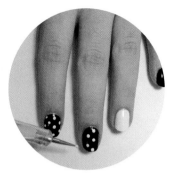

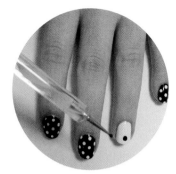

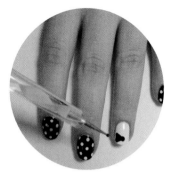

2 Using a dotting tool and a white nail polish, create a polka dot pattern on your black nails.

3 Using a dotting tool and the black nail polish, place a large black dot in the center of your white nails to be the knot of the bow.

4 Using a nail art brush and a black nail polish, create sideways heart shapes on each side of the black dot to be the loops of the bow.

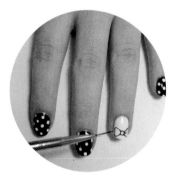

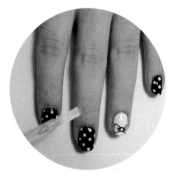

6 Using a nail art brush and the black nail polish, add detail to the bow by drawing a V-shape inside each loop.

7 Finally, apply a top coat to your nails to seal in the design.

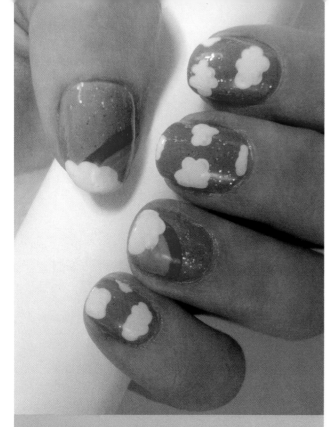

CLOUD AND RAINBOW NAILS

In need of a smile? Paint on this beautiful design for an even brighter day.

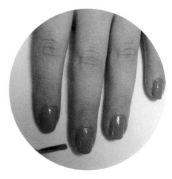

1 Start by painting your nails with a light pink nail polish.

5 Using a dotting tool and a white nail polish, make a few clusters of dots on every nail except the ring fingers. These will create clouds.

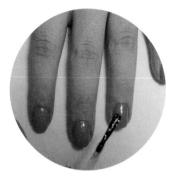

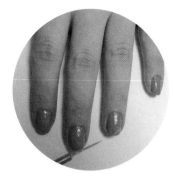

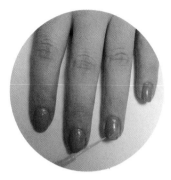

2 Apply a layer of rainbow glitter nail polish over the pink.

3 Using a nail art brush and a blue nail polish, create a curved line at the bottom right corner of your nail.

4 Repeat the previous step using the rest of the colors of this rainbow (green, yellow, red). The red arc will be the largest.

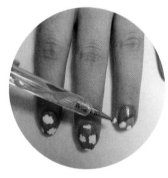

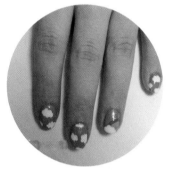

6 Using the same method, create a few clouds at the base of the rainbow.

7 Finally, apply a top coat to your nails to seal in the design.

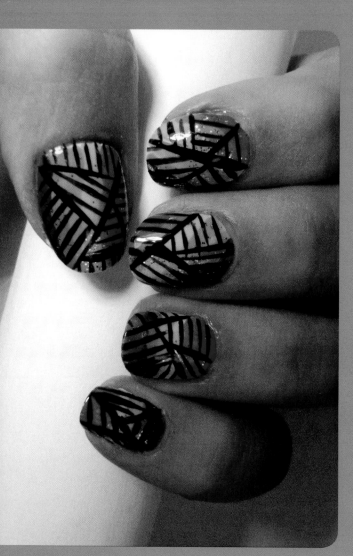

ABSTRACT OVER RAINBOW NAILS

A colorful rainbow shows through this fun abstract pattern.

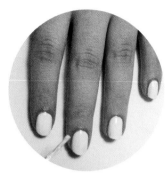

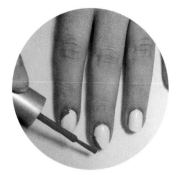

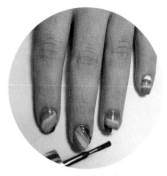

1 Start by painting your nails with a white nail polish.

2 Using a nail art brush and a red nail polish, paint a line starting at the edge of your nail.

3 Continue to add lines of nail color (orange, yellow, green, blue, and purple) to complete the rainbow.

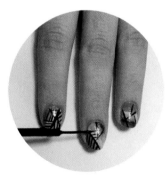

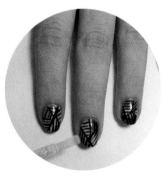

4 Using a nail art brush and a black nail polish, draw straight lines randomly across your nails.

5 Finally, apply a top coat to your nails to seal in the design.

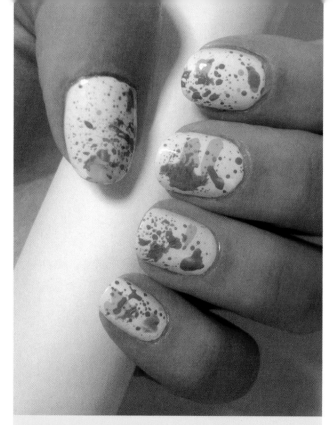

PAINT SPLATTER NAILS

A simple and easy-to-do nail art design with a funky spattered paint effect.

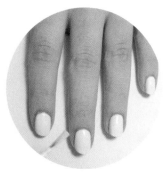

1 Start by painting your nails with a white nail polish.

4 Repeat these steps with pink and blue nail polishes.

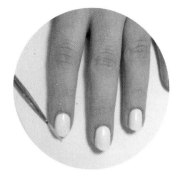

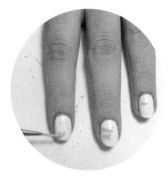

2 Protect your work surface by laying a piece of paper underneath your nails. Then mix a yellow nail polish with a nail polish thinner (or water, if you're using acrylic paint) and dip your nail art brush into the mixture. Tap the brush on the table and close to your nail so that the paint splatters onto the nail.

3 For bigger spots, dab the color on with the brush.

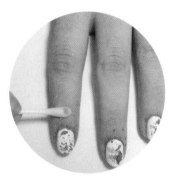

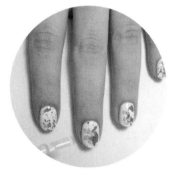

5 Using a Q-tip and acetone, remove any nail polish that landed on your skin.

6 Finally, apply a top coat to your nails to seal in the design.

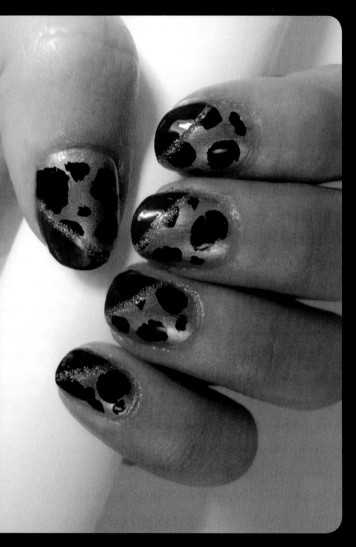

MAROON LEOPARD PRINT NAILS

A pop of color adds a fun flair to the original leopard print nails.

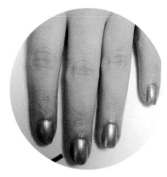

1 Start by painting your nails with a gold nail polish.

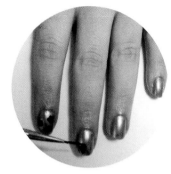

2 Using a nail art brush and brown nail polish, place spots all over your nails.

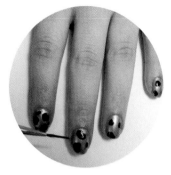

3 Using a nail art brush and a black nail polish, roughly outline the brown spots, adding a few spots of black in empty areas.

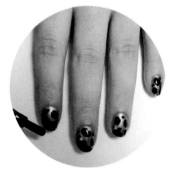

4 Using a nail art brush and a maroon nail polish, draw a diagonal line at the bottom of your nails.

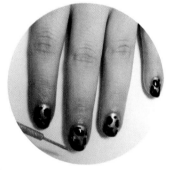

5 Add a line of gold glitter nail polish to the edge of the maroon.

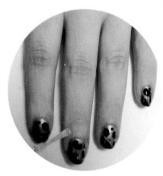

6 Finally, apply a top coat to your nails to seal in the design.

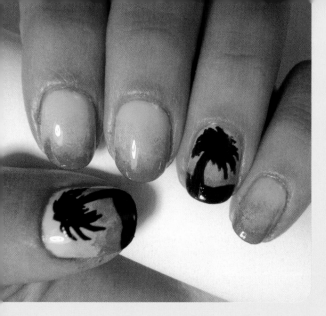

PALM TREE NAILS

This nail art features the beautiful silhouette of a palm tree in front of a summer sunset.

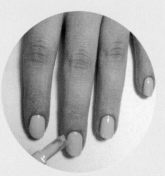

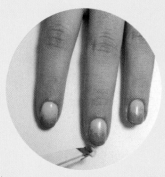

1 Start by painting your nails with a yellow nail polish.

2 Using a small piece of a cosmetic sponge and some tweezers, apply an orange nail polish to your nails. Leave the top third of your nails mostly yellow.

3 Dab on a hot pink nail polish using the same method, but this time focus on the tips of your nails.

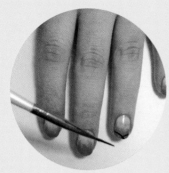

4 Using a nail art brush and a dark brown nail polish, create the silhouette of the beach by drawing two half circles on the tip of the nail.

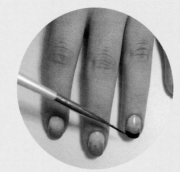

5 Using the same tool and nail polish, fill in the beach area completely.

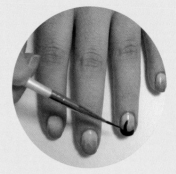

6 Using a nail art brush and a dark brown nail polish, create a curved line for the trunk of the tree. Thicken the bottom of the trunk.

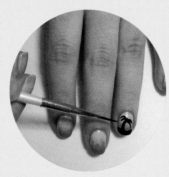

7 Using the same tool and nail polish, draw curved lines to create the leaves of the tree.

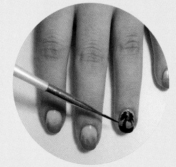

8 Go over the lines to thicken the leaves.

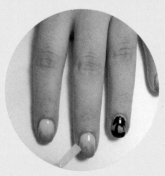

9 Finally, apply a top coat to your nails to seal in the design.

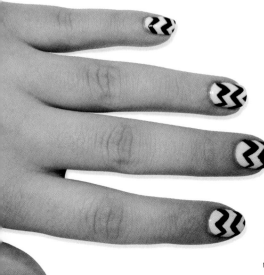

ZIGZAG NAILS

This eye-catching design will turn heads from across the room!

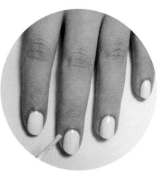

1 Start by painting your nails with a white nail polish.

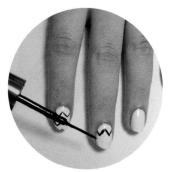

2 Using a nail art brush and a black nail polish, draw zigzag lines on all of your nails.

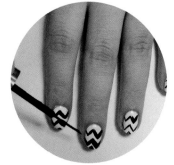

3 Thicken the lines to create an even look.

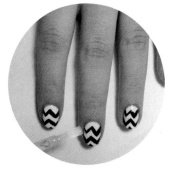

4 Finally, apply a top coat to your nails to seal in the design.

GIRAFFE PRINT NAILS

A classic giraffe print manicure.

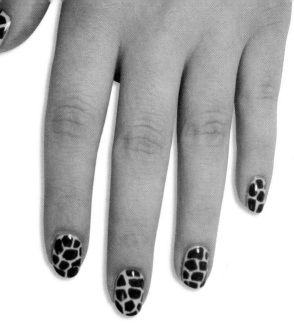

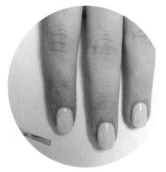

1 Start by painting your nails with a pale yellow nail polish.

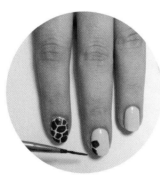

2 Using a nail art brush and a brown nail polish, create straight-edged rectangular shapes set closely together to form the giraffe print.

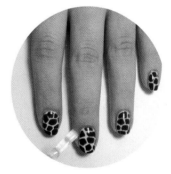

3 Finally, apply a top coat to your nails to seal in the design.

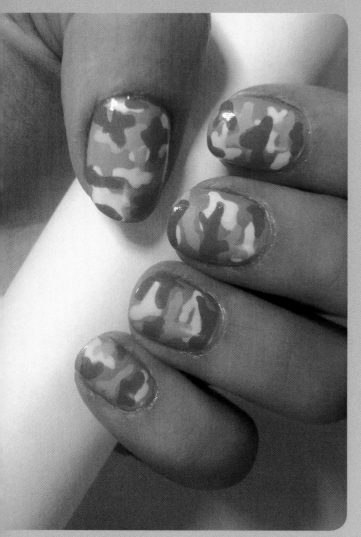

PINK CAMO NAILS

A cute and girly spin on camouflage.

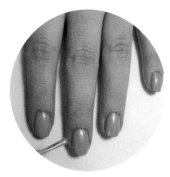

1   Start by painting your nails with a light pink nail polish.

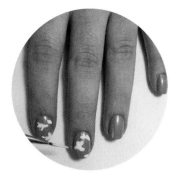

2   Using a nail art brush and a white nail polish, create irregular shapes all over your nails.

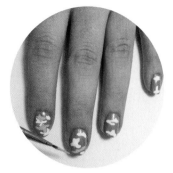

3   Repeat the previous step with a lighter pink nail polish. It's okay if the shapes overlap.

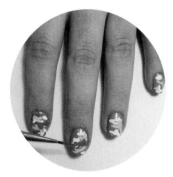

4   Repeat the step again with a darker pink nail polish.

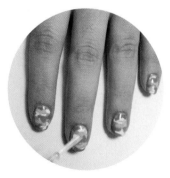

5   Finally, apply a top coat to your nails to seal in the design.

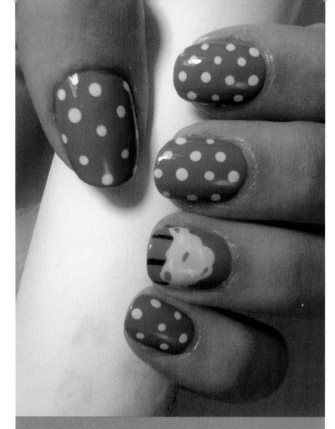

CUPCAKE NAILS

Bursting with sweetness and completely guilt-free, this yummy design is inspired by your favorite bakery treat!

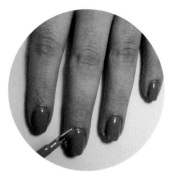

1 Start by painting your nails with a bright blue nail polish.

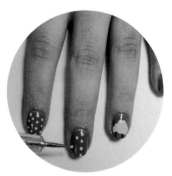

5 Using a dotting tool and the light pink nail polish, place small dots on the remaining nails.

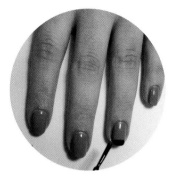
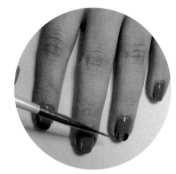
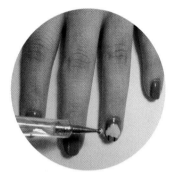

2 Using a nail art brush and a black nail polish, draw a thick horizontal line at the bottom of the ring finger nails. This will be the bottom of your cupcake.

3 Using a nail art brush and a brown nail polish, draw thick vertical lines within the black area.

4 Using a dotting tool and a light pink nail polish, place large dots in a pyramid shape on top of the cupcake. This will be the frosting on the cupcake.

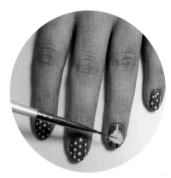
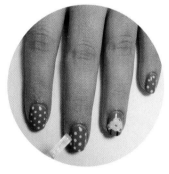

6 Using a nail art brush and a white nail polish, draw thin vertical lines on the frosting. Repeat this step using a bright pink nail polish. These will be the cupcake's sprinkles.

7 Finally, apply a top coat to your nails to seal in the design.

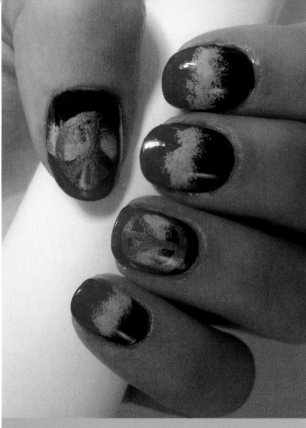

RASTAFARIAN NAILS

Take a trip down to Jamaica with nail art inspired by the Rastafarian movement.

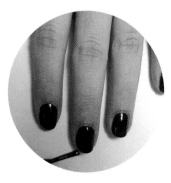

1   Start by painting your nails with a dark green nail polish.

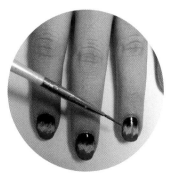

5   Using a nail art brush and a gold nail polish, draw a straight line down the center of the nail.

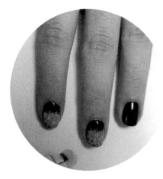

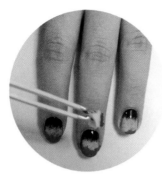

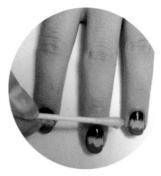

2 Using a small piece of a cosmetic sponge and some tweezers, apply a yellow nail polish to your nails. Leave the top third of your nails mostly dark green.

3 Dab on a red nail polish using the same method, but this time focus on the tips of your nails.

4 Using a Q-tip and acetone, remove any nail polish that landed on your skin.

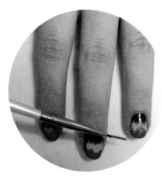

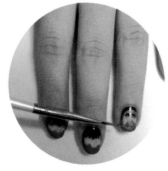

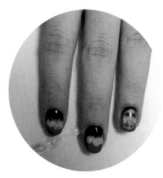

6 Using the same tool and nail polish, draw an inverted V-shape stemming from the bottom of the line you created.

7 Create a circle around it to form the basis of the peace symbol.

8 Finally, apply a top coat to your nails to seal in the design.

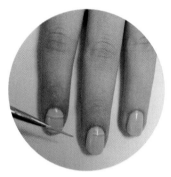

1 Start by painting your nails with a yellow nail polish. Using a nail art brush and a bright pink nail polish, create horizontal stripes of varying thicknesses on each of your nails.

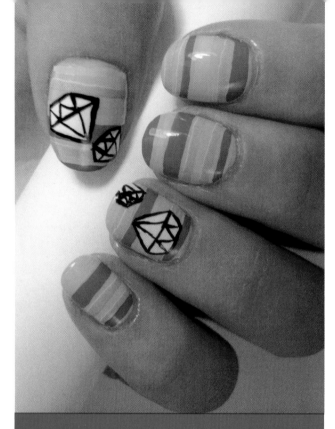

DIAMOND NAILS

Diamonds are a girl's best friend and with this bright, funky design you can show off their true sparkle.

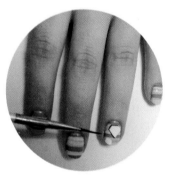

5 Using a nail art brush and a black nail polish, outline the white diamond.

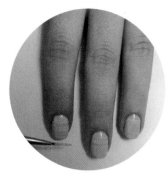 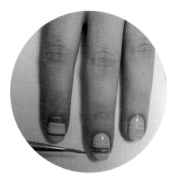 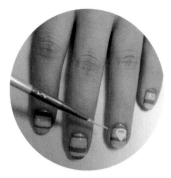

2 Using a nail art brush and a bright green nail polish, create more horizontal stripes on each of your nails.

3 Repeat the previous step with a bright blue nail polish.

4 Using a nail art brush and a white nail polish, draw a diamond shape in the center of the thumb and ring fingernails and fill it in.

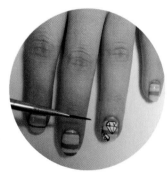 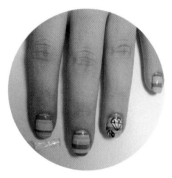

6 Using the same tool and nail polish, add details by creating lines and small triangles within the diamond to replicate the sides of the precious stone.

7 Finally, apply a top coat to your nails to seal in the design.

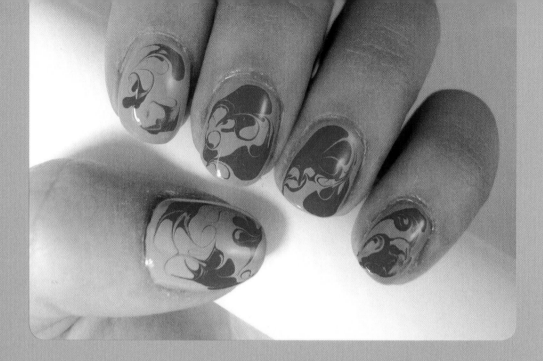

SWIRLED COLOR NAILS

This is an extremely easy and quick design that uses a technique called pin dragging. All you need are a few polishes and a needle or a pin. Change up the colors according to your taste. Be sure to only do one fingernail at a time; the technique is impossible to do otherwise.

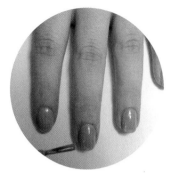

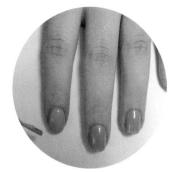

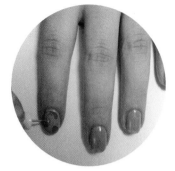

1 Start by painting your nails lightly with a turquoise blue nail polish.

2 Working on one nail at a time, paint on a thick layer of the turquoise.

3 Before the nail polish dries completely, quickly dot on a few spots of bright pink nail polish.

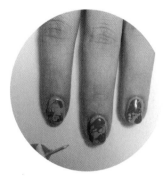

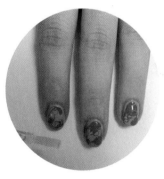

4 Using a pin, lightly swirl around the two colors in order to mix them. Don't overmix, or your design will become muddy.

5 Finally, apply a top coat to your nails to seal in the design.

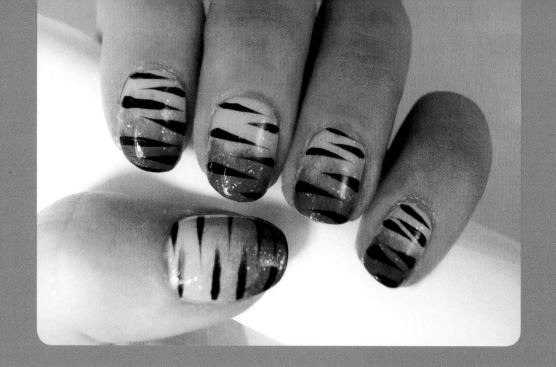

ORANGE AND PURPLE
TIGER PRINT NAILS

This design puts a spin on traditional animal
print with a gorgeous gradient effect.

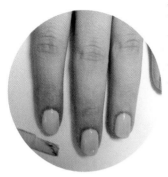

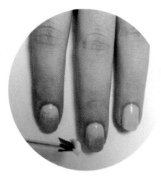

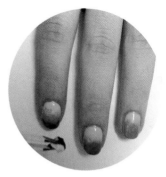

1 Start by painting your nails with a yellow nail polish.

2 Using a small piece of a cosmetic sponge and some tweezers, apply an orange nail polish to your nails. Leave the top third of your nails mostly yellow.

3 Dab on a purple nail polish using the same method, but this time focus on the tips of your nails.

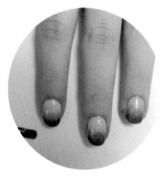

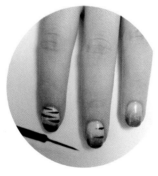

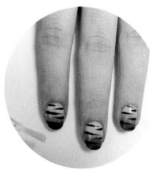

4 Apply a layer of multicolored glitter nail polish all over your nails.

5 Using a thin nail art brush and a black nail polish, create the tiger stripes starting from the sides of your nails going inwards.

6 Finally, apply a top coat to your nails to seal in the design.

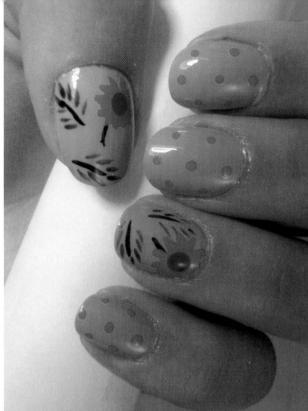

SIMPLE FLORAL NAILS

Another great design for those starting out, this fun floral pattern is inspired by spring.

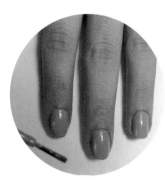

1 Start by painting your nails with a light blue nail polish.

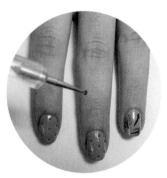

5 With a dotting tool and a red nail polish, make a dot for the center of the flower at the end of the stem.

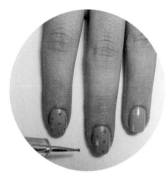

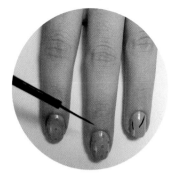

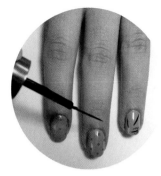

2 Using a dotting tool and a hot pink nail polish, make a polka dot pattern on all of your nails except the thumb and ring finger nails.

3 Using a nail art brush and a black nail polish, draw a few thin lines on the thumb and ring finger nails to be stems.

4 With a nail art brush and a green nail polish, create leaves by making short strokes along the black lines.

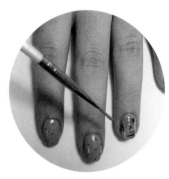

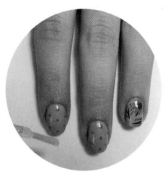

6 Using a nail art brush and a hot pink nail polish, create the flower petals by making short strokes radiating out from the center dot.

7 Finally, apply a top coat to your nails to seal in the design.

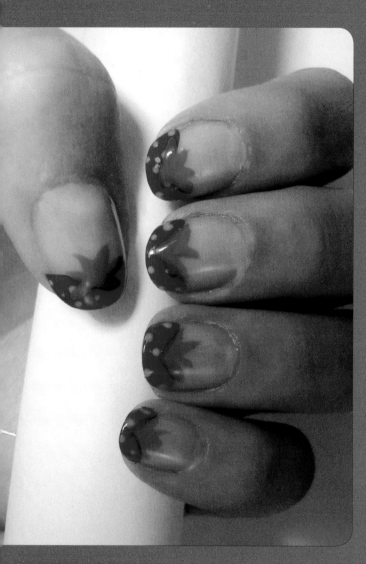

STRAWBERRY TIP NAILS

A fun twist on a French manicure, this design is cute enough for any season!

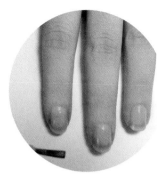

1 Start by painting your nails with a clear nail polish.

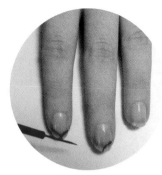

2 Using a nail art brush and a red nail polish, create a somewhat curved V-shape at the tips.

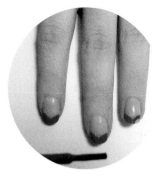

3 Using the same tool and nail polish, fill in the tips with red.

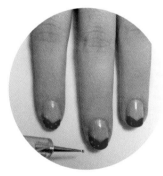

4 Using a dotting tool and a yellow nail polish, place small dots in the red area to make strawberry seeds.

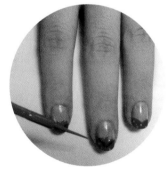

5 With a nail art brush and a green nail polish, create a few strokes above the strawberry to make the stem and leaves.

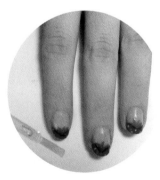

6 Finally, apply a top coat to your nails to seal in the design.

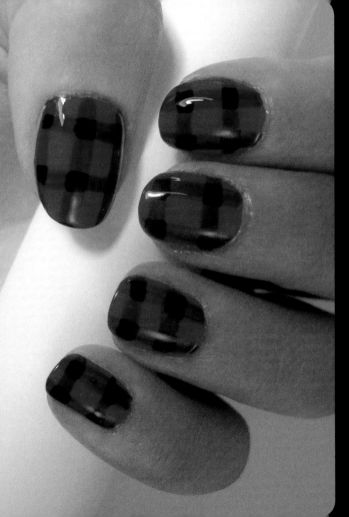

PLAID NAILS

This gorgeous plaid nail art design is a staple look. No matter what time of the year, it will always make a statement.

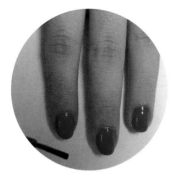

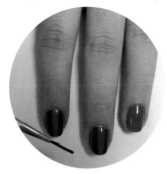

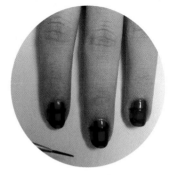

1 Start by painting your nails with a red nail polish.

2 Using a nail art brush and a dark red nail polish, draw thick vertical lines on your nails.

3 Using the same tool and nail polish, create horizontal lines crossing over the previous lines.

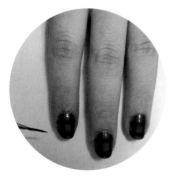

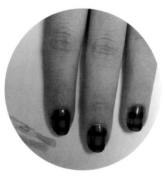

4 Using a nail art brush and a black nail polish, where the lines overlap, fill in the area with black.

5 Finally, apply a top coat to your nails to seal in the design.

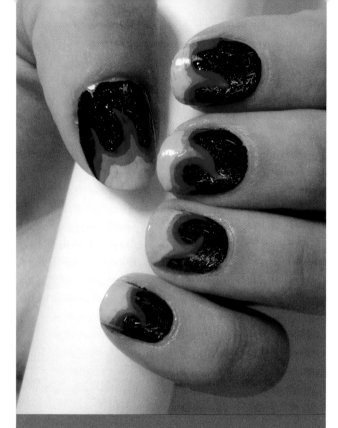

FIRE NAILS

....

Give your manicure an attitude with these fiery hot nails that are sure to grab attention.

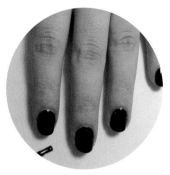

1 Start by painting your nails with a black nail polish.

5 Repeat Steps 3 and 4 with an orange nail polish, making the flame slightly smaller than the original one.

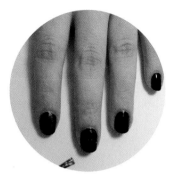

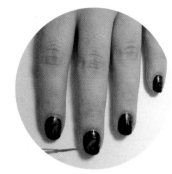

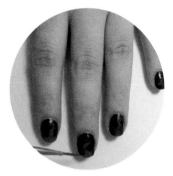

2 Apply a layer of gold glitter nail polish to your nails.

3 Using a nail art brush and a red nail polish, create a fire shape.

4 Using the same tool and nail polish, fill in the flame area.

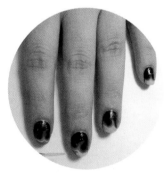

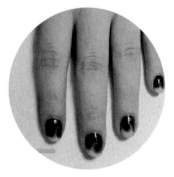

6 Using the same nail art brush and a yellow nail polish, create a fire shape within the orange area and fill in the flame area. This yellow flame will be the smallest.

7 Finally, apply a top coat to your nails to seal in the design.

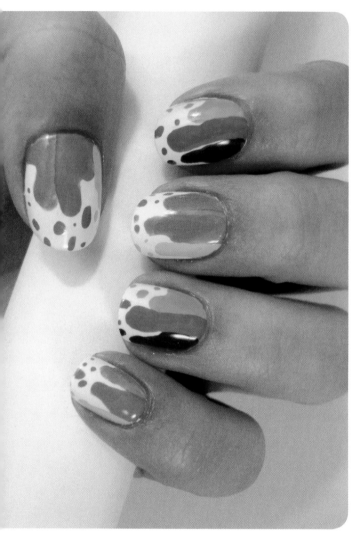

RAINBOW DRIP NAILS

Fulfill your artistic side and try this art-inspired manicure that looks like paint dripping down a canvas.

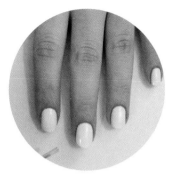

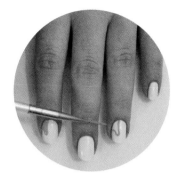

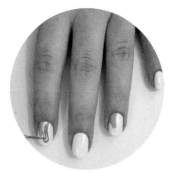

1 Start by painting your nails with a white nail polish.

2 Using a nail art brush and a green nail polish, create a drip along your nails. There's no wrong way to create a drip or recreate this design, so just have fun with it.

3 Using a nail art brush and a blue nail polish, create another drip along your nails.

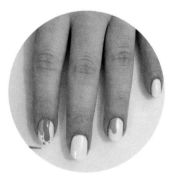

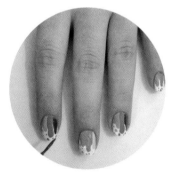

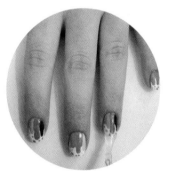

4 Using the same tool and nail polish, add a few spots of color below the drip shape to add a splatter effect.

5 Repeat Steps 2, 3, and 4 for the remaining colors (pink, orange, yellow, and purple).

6 Finally, apply a top coat to your nails to seal in the design.

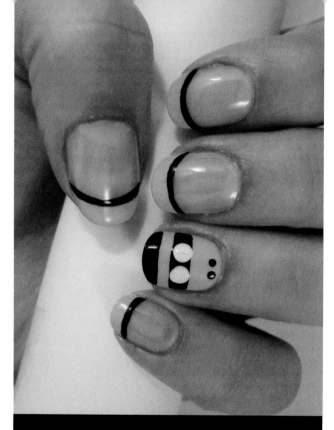

BUMBLEBEE NAILS

Bees are not usually something you would want anywhere near you, but in this case they are just too cute.

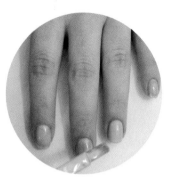

1 Start by painting your ring finger nails with a yellow nail polish.

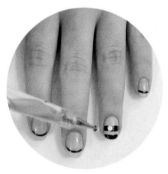

5 Using a dotting tool and a white nail polish, place dots on either side of the nail to create the wings of the bee.

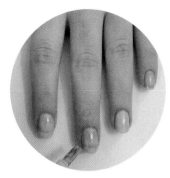

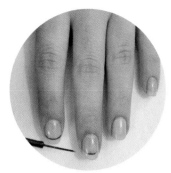

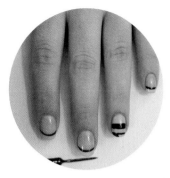

2 Paint the tips of the rest of your nails with the nail polish as if you were giving yourself a French manicure.

3 Using a thin nail art brush and a black nail polish, create a black line along the French tips.

4 Using a nail art brush and the black nail polish, create thick horizontal stripes on the ring finger, leaving a bit of space at the top for the bee's eyes.

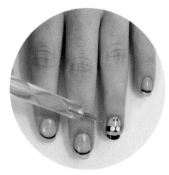

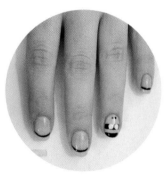

6 Using the same tool and a black nail polish, place two tiny dots above the stripes for the eyes.

7 Finally, apply a top coat to your nails to seal in the design.

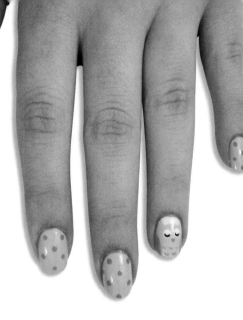

OWL NAILS

Shh! Don't wake the adorable sleeping owl in this polka dot design.

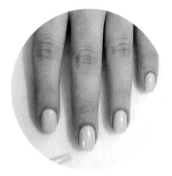

1 Start by painting your nails with a mint green nail polish.

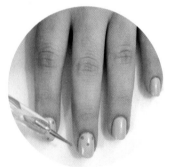

2 Using a dotting tool and a lime green nail polish, make a polka dot design on all of your nails except the ring finger, which will be saved for the owl design.

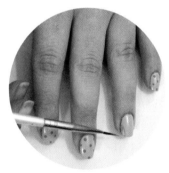

3 Using a nail art brush and a lime green nail polish, draw a half-moon shape on both sides of the ring finger. These will be the owl's wings.

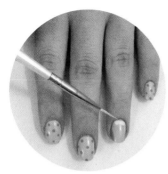

4 Using a nail art brush and a white nail polish, draw a rectangular shape at the top of your nail.

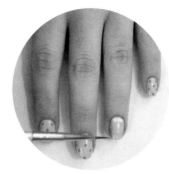

5 Using a nail art brush and a lime green nail polish, draw small curved lines in between the owl's wings. These will be his feathers.

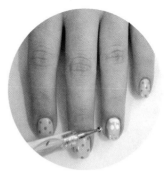

6 Using a dotting tool and a white nail polish, place two large dots underneath the white rectangle at the top of your nail.

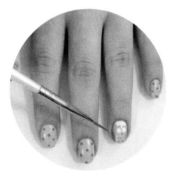

7 Using a nail art brush and an orange nail polish, create a tiny triangle for the beak.

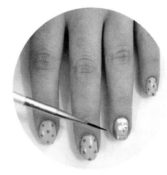

8 Using a thin nail art brush and the black nail polish, place two black curved lines inside the white eyes, to make it appear as if the owl's eyes are closed.

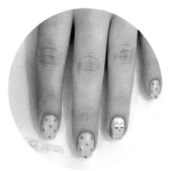

9 Finally, apply a top coat to your nails to seal in the design.

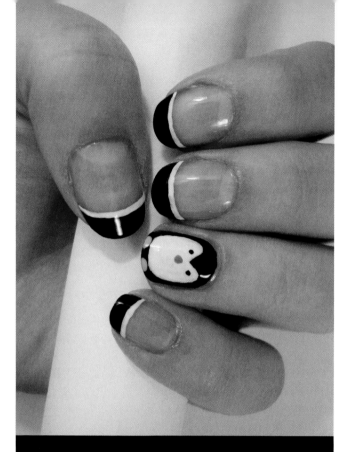

CUTE PENGUIN NAILS

....

This heartwarming manicure is great for the wintertime, or anytime, if you love penguins.

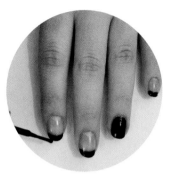

1 Using a nail art brush and a black nail polish, paint the tips of all your fingernails except your ring finger nails. Paint your ring finger nails completely with the black nail polish.

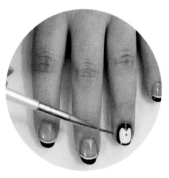

5 Using a nail art brush and an orange nail polish, make a small dot in the middle of the body for the beak.

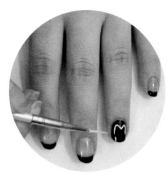

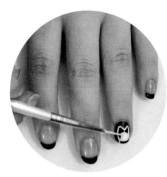

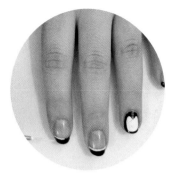

2 Using a nail art brush and a white nail polish, draw an M-shape in the middle of your ring finger nail.

3 Using the same tool and nail polish, draw a curved line at the bottom of the M-shape and fill in the area with white. This will be the penguin's body.

4 Using the same tool and nail polish, outline the top of your French tips.

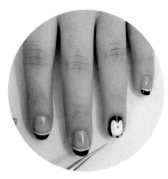

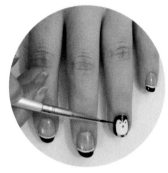

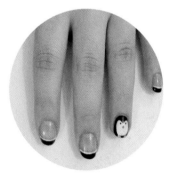

6 Using the same tool and a yellow nail polish, place two larger dots on the sides of the body by the base of the nail for the penguin's feet.

7 Using a thin nail art brush and the black nail polish, place a tiny dot on either side of the beak for the eyes.

8 Finally, apply a top coat to your nails to seal in the design.

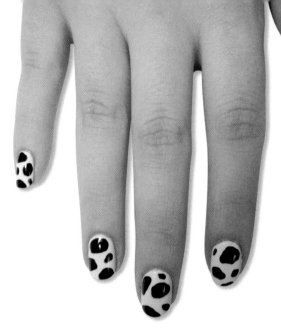

COW PRINT NAILS

A cow print can be super cute! Show off your country side with this simple manicure.

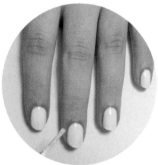

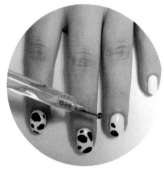

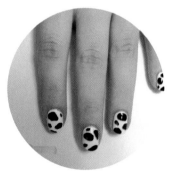

1 Start by painting your nails with a white nail polish.

2 Using a dotting tool and a black nail polish, create irregular dots all over your nails to be the cow spots. It may help to look at a photo of the print to get the best design.

3 Finally, apply a top coat to your nails to seal in the design.

RUBBER DUCKY NAILS

An extremely cute design, you'll love showing off your new bathtub friend!

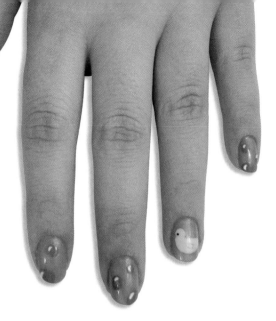

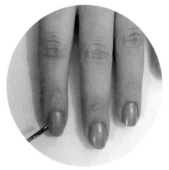

1 Start by painting your nails with a light pink nail polish.

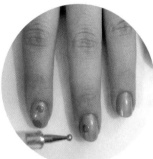

2 Using a dotting tool and a blue nail polish, create various sizes of dots on all your nails except the ring fingers. These will be soap bubbles.

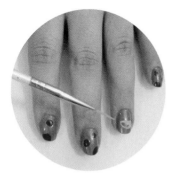

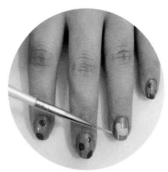

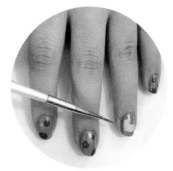

3 Using a nail art brush and a yellow nail polish, create a half-circle shape on the ring finger nail.

4 Using the same tool and nail polish, draw a circle for the duck's head on one side of the half circle.

5 Using a nail art brush and an orange nail polish, draw the beak sticking out of the head.

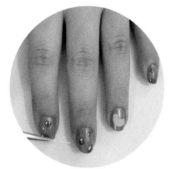

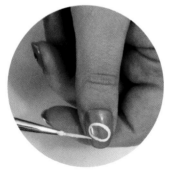

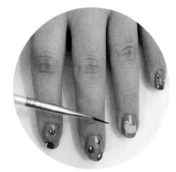

6 With a nail art brush and the white nail polish, add a small curved line to the bubbles to suggest a shine.

7 With the same tool and nail polish, create a large oval for a bar of soap on the thumbnail.

8 Using a dotting tool and a black nail polish, place a small black dot on the duck's head to make an eye.

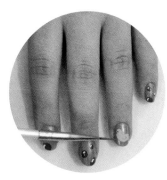

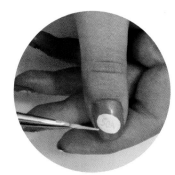

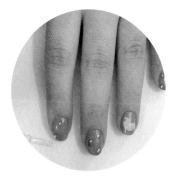

9 Using the same tool and the orange nail polish, add the outline of a wing in the center of the body.

10 Using a nail art brush and a gray nail polish, write "Soap" on the bar of soap you created on your thumbs.

11 Finally, apply a top coat to your nails to seal in the design.

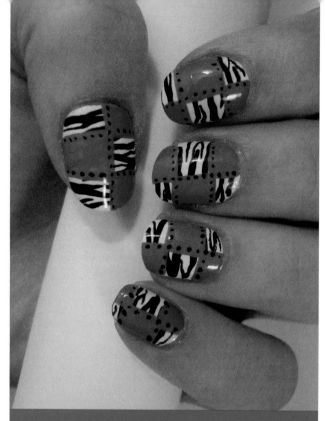

BLUE AND ZEBRA CHECKERED NAILS

A unique nail design incorporates both a checkered pattern and a fun zebra print.

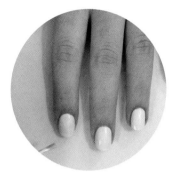

1 Start by painting your nails with a white nail polish.

5 Using a nail art brush and the blue nail polish, fill in every other square with blue.

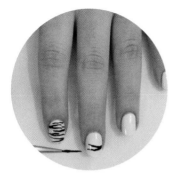

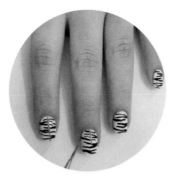

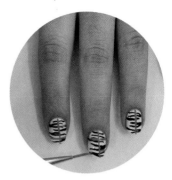

2 Using a thin nail art brush and a black nail polish, create a zebra print by making wavy lines side to side along your nails. Make sure that the waves go in both directions.

3 Using a nail art brush and a blue nail polish, draw a straight line down the middle of the nail.

4 Using the same tool and nail polish, draw two horizontal lines across the vertical line you just created, evenly spaced apart.

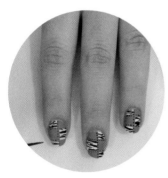

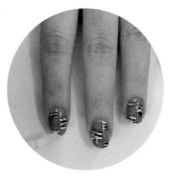

6 Using a nail art brush and the black nail polish, place dots along the outline of the squares.

7 Finally, apply a top coat to your nails to seal in the design.

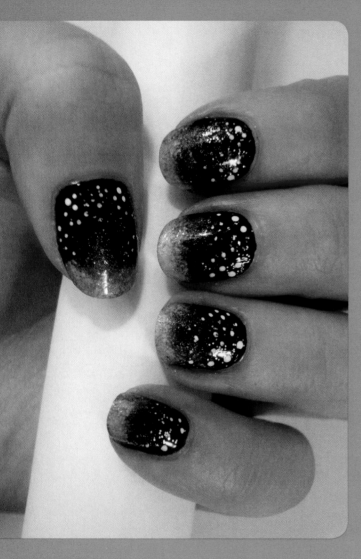

STARRY SKY NAILS

You don't have to wish on a shooting star to create dreamy nails. With this simple design, you'll light up the sky in no time!

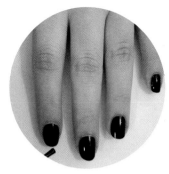

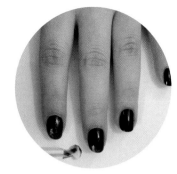

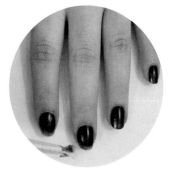

1 Start by painting your nails with a black nail polish.

2 Using a small piece of a cosmetic sponge and some tweezers, apply a sparkly blue nail polish to your nails. Leave the top third of your nails mostly black.

3 Dab on a light blue nail polish using the same method, but this time focus on the tips of your nails.

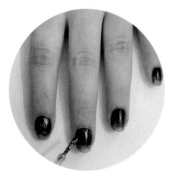

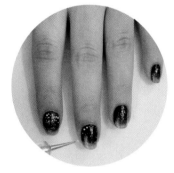

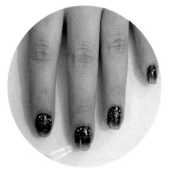

4 Apply a silver glitter to the entire surface of all of your nails to help blend the two colors together.

5 Using a dotting tool and a white nail polish, create very small dots at the top of your nails. These will be the stars in your night sky.

6 Finally, apply a top coat to your nails to seal in the design.

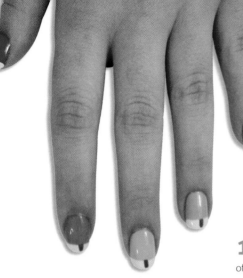

ICE CREAM POP NAILS

A summer manicure that will satisfy the biggest sweet tooth.

1 Start by painting each of your nails with brightly colored nail polishes.

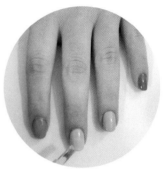

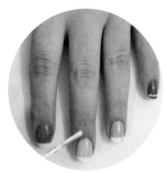

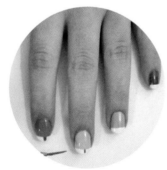

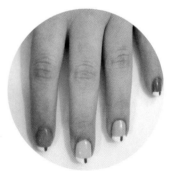

2 Using a thin nail art brush and a white nail polish, paint the tips of your nails. This will look exactly like a brightly colored French manicure.

3 Using a nail art brush and a dark orange nail polish, draw a long, thin oval shape in the center of your tips to make the pop's stick.

4 Finally, apply a top coat to your nails to seal in the design.

PINK SKULL NAILS

Add a little rock 'n' roll to your nails with this edgy, but girly, nail design.

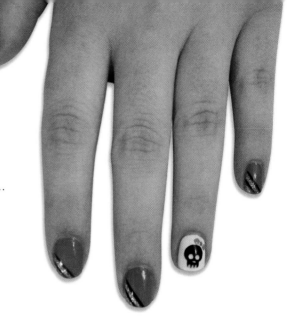

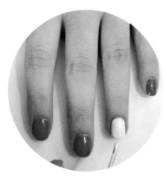

1 Start by painting your ring finger nails with a white nail polish. Paint the rest of your nails with a hot pink nail polish.

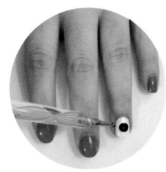

2 Using a dotting tool and a black nail polish, create a large oval shape on your ring finger nails. This will be the skull.

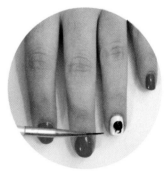

3 Using a nail art brush and the same nail polish, add a small horizontal black rectangle below the oval for the jaw.

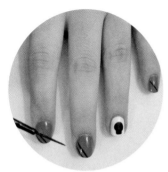

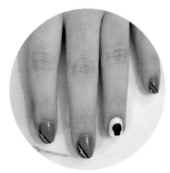

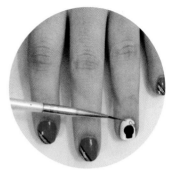

4 Using the same tool and nail polish, draw two black diagonal lines across the other nails.

5 Using a nail art brush and a silver glitter nail polish, paint a line between the two black lines.

6 Using a nail art brush and a light pink nail polish, draw an infinity symbol on the side of the skull and fill it in. This will be the skull's bow.

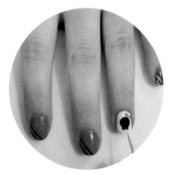

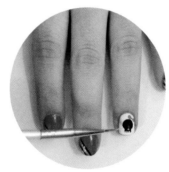

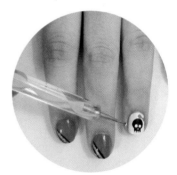

7 Using a nail art brush and the white nail polish, add teeth to the jaw using short strokes.

8 Using the same tool and nail polish, place a small white horizontal line in the center of the skull for the nose.

9 Using a dotting tool and the white nail polish, add two dots for the eyes.

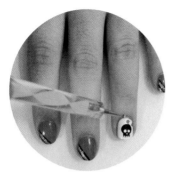 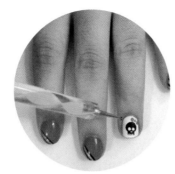 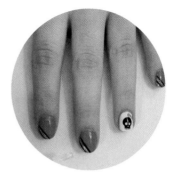

10 Using a dotting tool and the white nail polish, make a large white dot for the knot of the bow.

11 Using the dotting tool and the pink nail polish, place a smaller pink dot inside it.

12 Finally, apply a top coat to your nails to seal in the design.

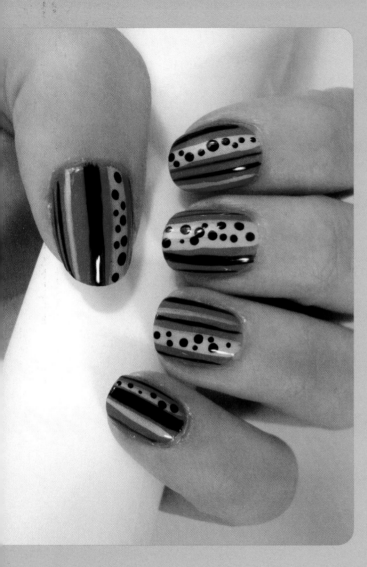

BLACK AND PINK STRIPE NAILS

Great for beginners, this design is a quick and simple look for anyone.

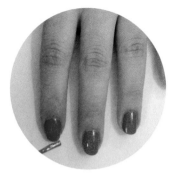 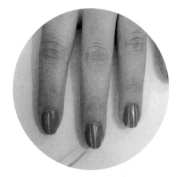 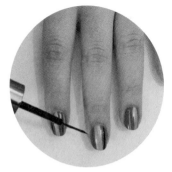

1 Start by painting your nails with a hot pink nail polish.

2 Using a nail art brush and a light pink nail polish, draw vertical lines of varying thicknesses.

3 Repeat Step 2 with a black nail polish.

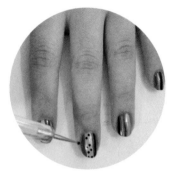 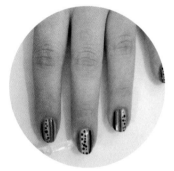

4 Using a dotting tool and the black nail polish, place a few dots in the thicker lines.

5 Finally, apply a top coat to your nails to seal in the design.

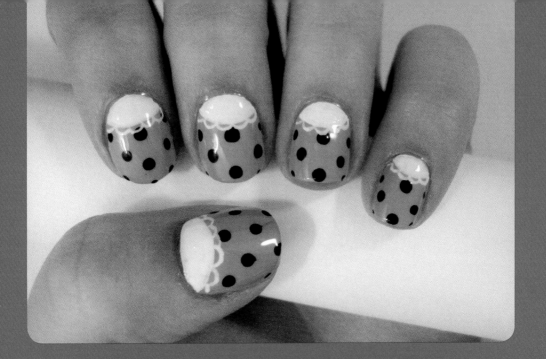

TURQUOISE AND BROWN NAILS

This classic design combines the elegance of lace with the simplicity of polka dots.

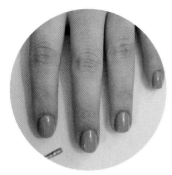

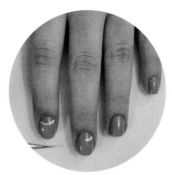

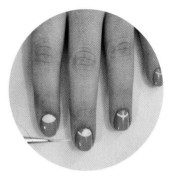

1 Start by painting your nails with a turquoise nail polish.

2 Using a nail art brush and a white nail polish, create a half-moon shape at the base of your nails.

3 Fill in the half-moon area completely with white nail polish.

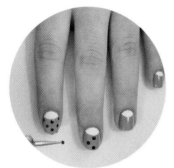

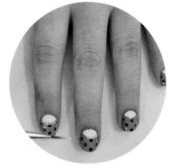

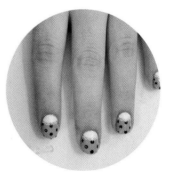

4 Using a dotting tool and a brown nail polish, place dots in the remaining blue area.

5 Using a nail art brush and the white nail polish, place loops along the edge of the white half-moon shape to create a lace pattern.

6 Finally, apply a top coat to your nails to seal in the design.

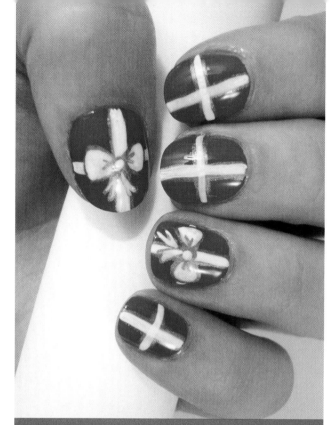

GIFT-WRAPPED NAILS

A lovely manicure inspired by the beautifully wrapped gifts under the Christmas tree.

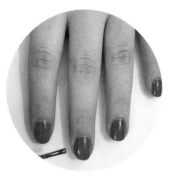

1 Start by painting your nails with a red nail polish.

5 Using the same tool and nail polish, create the loops of the bow by painting a curve on each side of the X-shape. Fill in the resulting loops completely with gold.

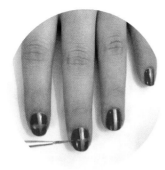

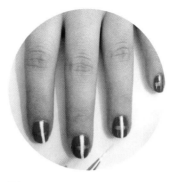

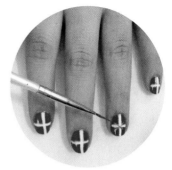

2 Using a nail art brush and a gold nail polish, paint a cross on your nails.

3 Using a nail art brush and a white nail polish, paint a thinner white line inside the gold line.

4 Using a nail art brush and the gold nail polish, begin the bow by painting an X-shape in the center of the ring finger and thumb nails.

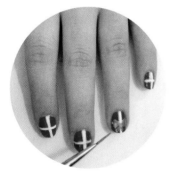

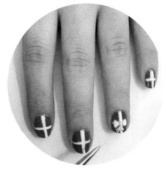

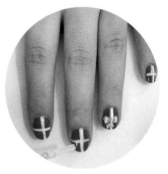

6 Using the same tool and nail polish, draw the ends of the ribbon extending down from the knot, ending them in a V-shaped notch. Fill in the ends completely with gold.

7 Using a nail art brush and the white nail polish, fill in the bow, leaving an outline of gold.

8 Finally, apply a top coat to your nails to seal in the design.

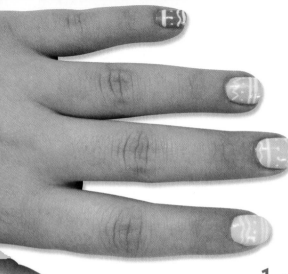

EASTER EGG NAILS

Why wait until Easter to decorate eggs? With this cute nail design, you can decorate your nails with your favorite Easter egg creations!

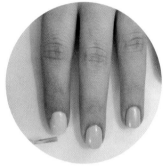

1 Start by painting each of your nails with pastel nail polishes.

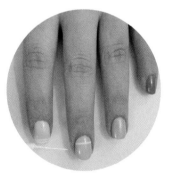

2 Using a thin nail art brush and a white nail polish, draw straight lines across your nails.

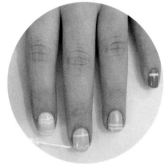

3 Using the same tool and nail polish, add wavy lines, zigzag lines, and dots between the straight lines.

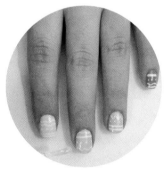

4 Finally, apply a top coat to your nails to seal in the design.

SUMMER FRUIT NAILS

Bring the best part of summer to your nails with these super-cute fruit designs.

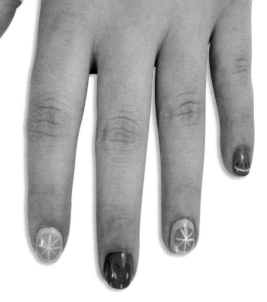

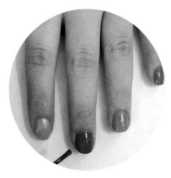

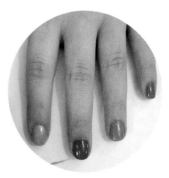

1 Start by painting your thumbnails with a light yellow nail polish. Paint one of each of the rest of your nails with medium yellow, red, light orange, and pink nail polish.

2 Using a nail art brush and the yellow nail polish, place small dots on your red nails. These will be strawberries.

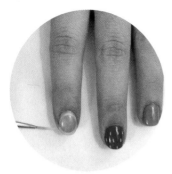 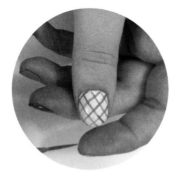 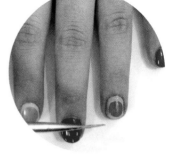

3 Using the same tool and nail polish, create the outline of a circle on your medium yellow nail, and fill it in. This will be a slice of citrus fruit.

4 Using a nail art brush and a light brown nail polish, draw a crisscross pattern on your thumbnails. These will be pineapples.

5 Using the same tool and a dark orange nail polish, create the outline of a circle on your light orange nail, and fill it in. This will be an orange wedge.

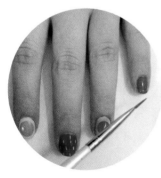 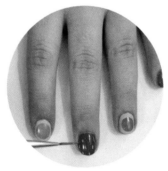 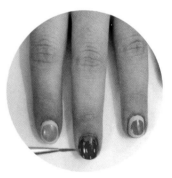

6 Using a nail art brush and a green nail polish, add a green French tip to your pink nails. These will be slices of watermelon.

7 Using the same tool and nail polish, draw a zigzag across the top of your red nails to make leaves for your strawberries.

8 Fill in the strawberry leaves with the green.

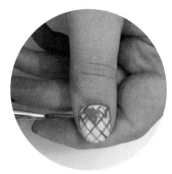

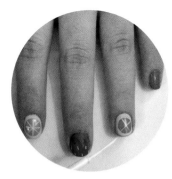

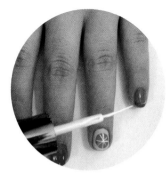

9 Using a nail art brush and the green nail polish, draw another zigzag across the top of your thumbnails to add leaves to your pineapples. Fill in the area with the green.

10 Using the same tool and a white nail polish, add lines inside the medium yellow and orange nails to create the wedges.

11 Using the same tool and nail polish, draw a line of white along the inner edge of the green tip.

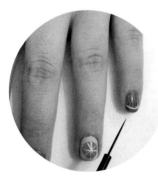

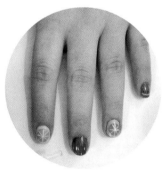

12 Using a small dotting tool and a black nail polish, add black seeds along the French tip.

13 Finally, apply a top coat to your nails to seal in the design.

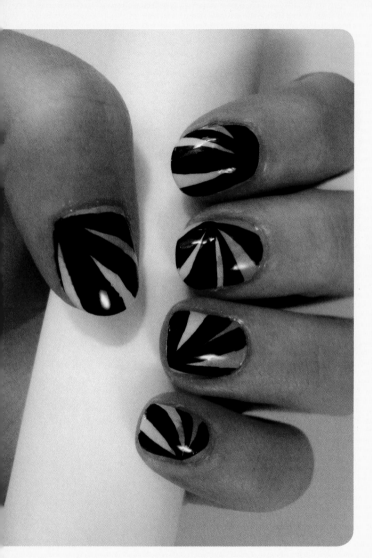

LIGHT BURST
NAILS

Bright pastel colors peek out
of a black abstract design in
this light-burst nail art.

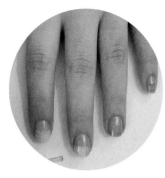

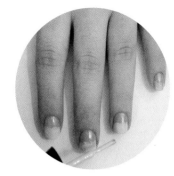

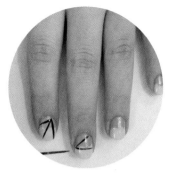

1 Start by painting the top half of your nails with a light pink nail polish. Paint the bottom half of your nails with a pale yellow nail polish.

2 Add more layers of the light pink and pale yellow nail polishes to fade the two colors into each other.

3 Using a nail art brush and a black nail polish, create a fan shape out of black lines. The lines can stem from any corner of your nail.

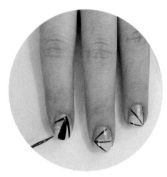

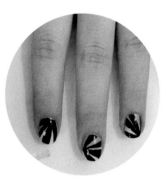

4 Thicken the ends of the black lines with more layers of nail polish.

5 Finally, apply a top coat to your nails to seal in the design.

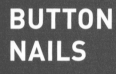

BUTTON NAILS

Make sure your nails are as cute as a button with this charming nail art design.

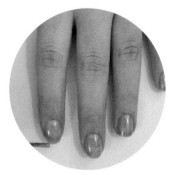

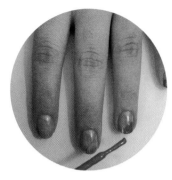

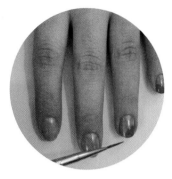

1 Using a pale blue nail polish, create half circles on the tips of your thumb, index finger, and middle finger nails.

2 Using a pink nail polish, create half circles on the tips of your ring finger and little finger nails.

3 With a nail art brush and a darker red nail polish, draw the outline of a smaller circle inside each of the circles on your ring finger and little finger nails. Add two short strokes for button holes.

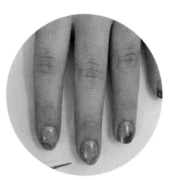

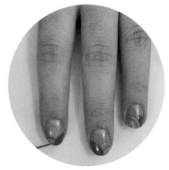

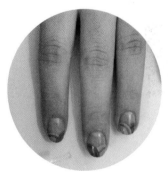

4 Repeat the previous step with a darker blue nail polish and your thumb, index finger, and middle finger nails.

5 Following the previous steps, alternate the pink and blue nail polishes to create overlapping buttons.

6 Finally, apply a top coat to your nails to seal in the design.

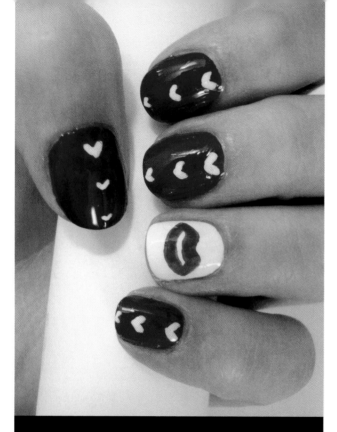

LIPS THEME NAILS

With this fun nail design, you won't have to steal kisses on Valentine's Day.

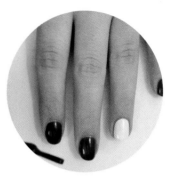

1 Start by painting your ring finger nails with a white nail polish. Paint the rest of your nails with a dark red nail polish.

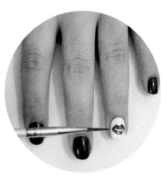

5 Using a nail art brush and the red nail polish, fill in each part of the lip.

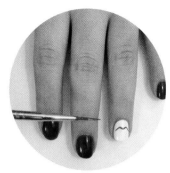

2   Using a nail art brush and a red nail polish, draw a rounded M-shape on your ring finger nails to make the top of the lips.

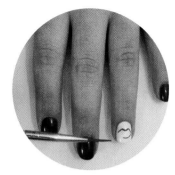

3   Using the same tool and nail polish, connect the bottom of the M-shape with a curved line to make the bottom of the lips.

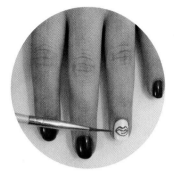

4   Using the same tool and nail polish, add a smaller M-shape and curved line inside the lips.

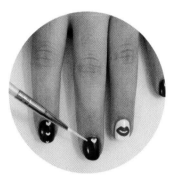

6   Using a nail art brush and a white nail polish, create hearts by drawing little rounded V-shapes on the rest of your nails.

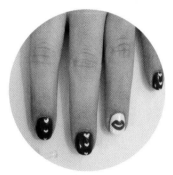

7   Finally, apply a top coat to your nails to seal in the design.

SILVER GLITTER HEART NAILS

Another great design for beginners! These simple silver hearts will stand out and make your nails shine.

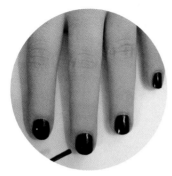

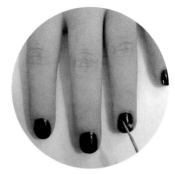

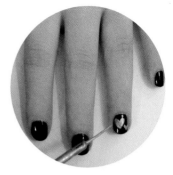

1 Start by painting your nails with a black nail polish.

2 Using a nail art brush and a silver nail polish, create a small V-shape, or heart, on the lower right corners of your thumb and ring finger nails.

3 Using the same tool and nail polish, create a bigger V-shape, or heart, on the upper left corners of your thumb and ring finger nails.

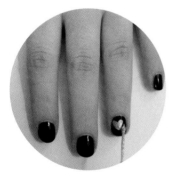

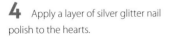

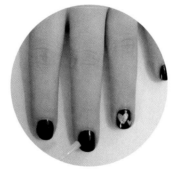

4 Apply a layer of silver glitter nail polish to the hearts.

5 Finally, apply a top coat to your nails to seal in the design.

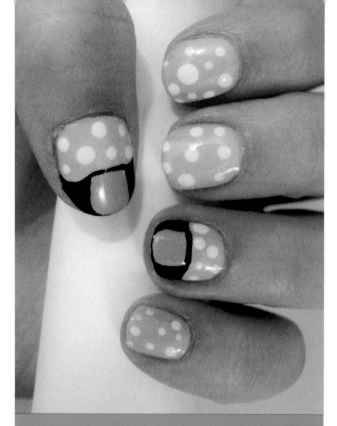

MUSHROOM NAILS

With these nails inspired by the forest, you will be able to bring the outdoors with you wherever you go.

1 Start by painting your nails with a light blue nail polish.

5 Using a dotting tool and a white nail polish, place dots on the top of the mushroom.

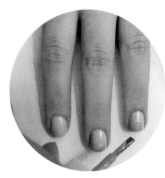

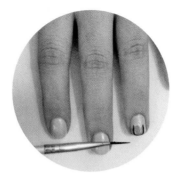

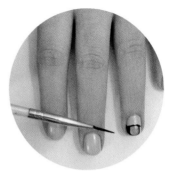

2 Using a nail art brush and a light brown nail polish, draw a thick vertical line at the bottom of the ring finger and thumb nails. This will be the stem of the mushroom.

3 Using a nail art brush and a black nail polish, outline the stem.

4 Using a nail art brush and the black nail polish, draw the top of the mushroom and fill in the background with black.

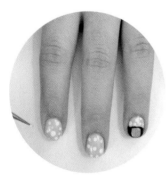

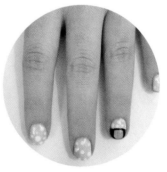

6 Place white dots on the remaining nails.

7 Finally, apply a top coat to your nails to seal in the design.

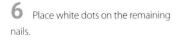

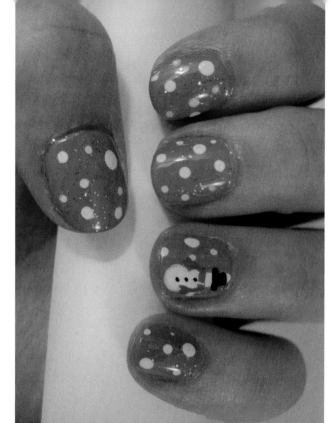

SNOWMAN NAILS

Show off this cute snowman manicure during the snowy season.

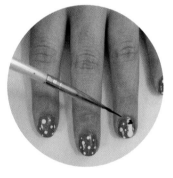

1 Start by painting your nails with a glittery lilac nail polish.

5 Using the same tool and nail polish, add a black square above the line to form your snowman's hat.

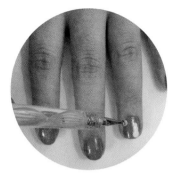

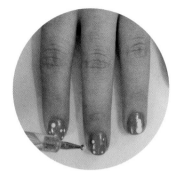

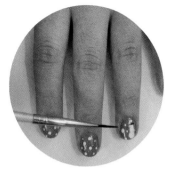

2 Using a dotting tool and a white nail polish, place a large dot at the bottom of your ring finger nails, then a medium-sized dot above it, and a small one to top it all off. This will be your snowman.

3 Using the same tool and nail polish, place random white dots of various sizes for the snowflakes on the other nails.

4 Using a nail art brush and a black nail polish, draw a thick black horizontal line above the head of your snowman.

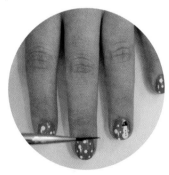

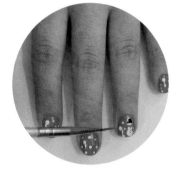

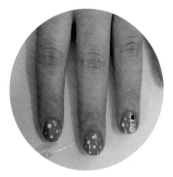

6 Using the same tool and nail polish, give your snowman buttons by placing a few dots down the middle of the two bottom white dots.

7 Using a nail art brush and a blue nail polish, draw a line across your snowman's neck and down to his side for a scarf.

8 Finally, apply a top coat to your nails to seal in the design.

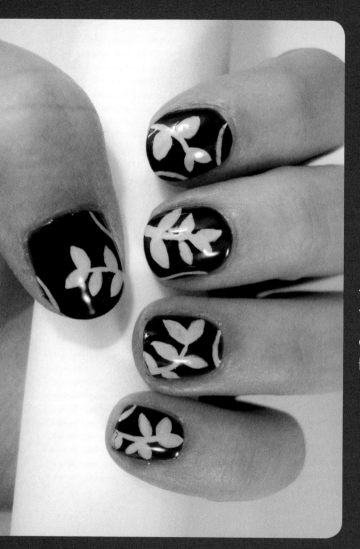

PURPLE
LEAVES NAILS

....

You'll warm up to the
changing season with these
fall-inspired nails.

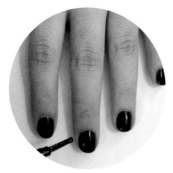

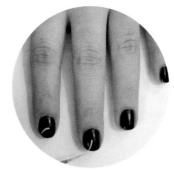

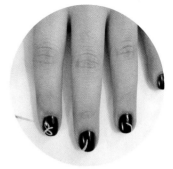

1 Start by painting your nails with a dark purple nail polish.

2 Using a nail art brush and a lilac nail polish, draw curved lines on your nails. These will be the stems of the leaves.

3 Using the same tool and nail polish, start at the stems and draw oval leaf shapes. Fill them in with lilac.

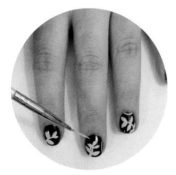

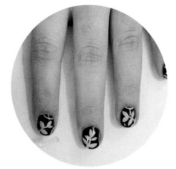

4 Using the nail art brush and the lilac nail polish, feel free to add a few more stems in the empty space around the leaves on your nails.

5 Finally, apply a top coat to your nails to seal in the design.

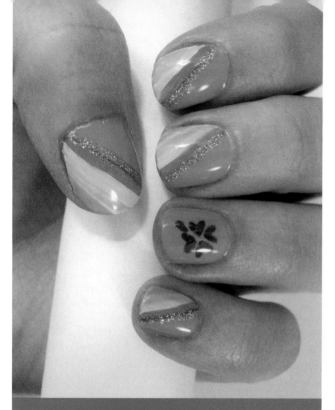

ST. PATRICK'S DAY NAILS

Forget those boring green shirts and have some fun this St. Patrick's Day with this rainbow and clover nail art.

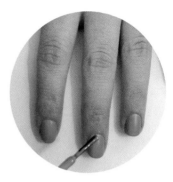

1 Start by painting your nails with a green nail polish.

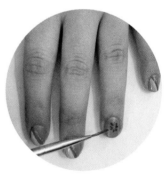

5 Using a nail art brush and a dark green nail polish, draw four heart-shaped leaves stemming from a central point on your ring finger nail. This will be a four-leaf clover.

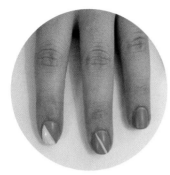

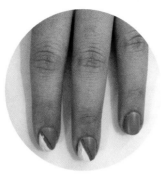

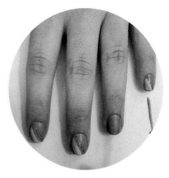

2 Using a nail art brush and a white nail polish, draw a diagonal across each of your nails except for the ring finger. Fill in the left side of the diagonal with the white polish.

3 Using a thin nail art brush and a pink nail polish, draw another diagonal along the outside of the first one. This is the beginning of the rainbow.

4 Repeat this using the colors yellow, green, and blue. The blue will be the smallest arc. Using a nail art brush and a gold glitter nail polish, outline your rainbow along the outer edge next to the pink arc.

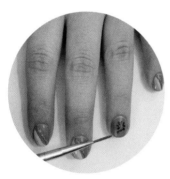

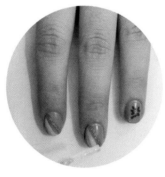

6 Using a nail art brush and the green nail polish, draw a triangular shape at the bottom four-leaf clover for the stem.

7 Finally, apply a top coat to your nails to seal in the design.

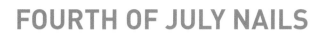

FOURTH OF JULY NAILS

Show your patriotism on July 4th with these red, white, and blue nails.

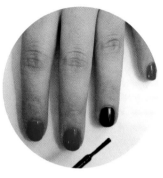

1 Start by painting your ring finger nails with a blue nail polish. Paint the rest of your nails with a red nail polish.

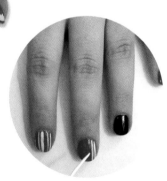

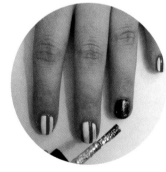

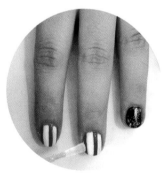

2 Using a thin nail art brush and a white nail polish, draw horizontal lines on the red nails. Go over the lines a few times to thicken them. These stripes represent the ones on the American flag.

3 For stars, apply a chunky silver glitter nail polish to your blue nails.

4 Finally, apply a top coat to your nails to seal in the design.

SPORTS NAILS

Whether you are a sports fanatic or just want to show off one sport as an accent nail, this design featuring a basketball, a baseball, a tennis ball, a football, and a soccer ball is for you.

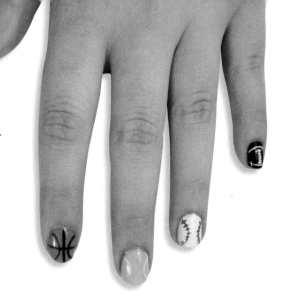

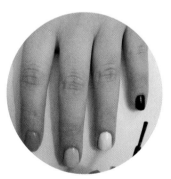

1 Start by painting each of your nails with a different color nail polish to represent each ball: an orange nail polish for the basketball, a white nail polish for the baseball, a yellow nail polish for the tennis ball, a dark brown nail polish for the football, and a white nail polish for the soccer ball.

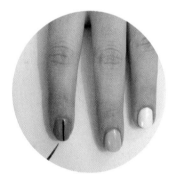

2 For the basketball nail: Using a nail art brush and a black nail polish, draw a vertical line down the center of the orange nail.

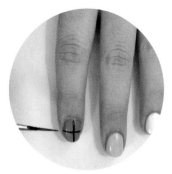 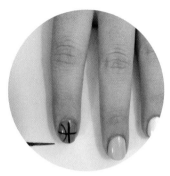 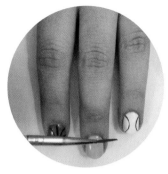

3 Using the same tool and nail polish, draw a black horizontal line across the middle of the nail, bisecting the vertical line.

4 Using the same tool and nail polish, draw two black lines curving inward, one on each side of the nail.

5 For the baseball nail: Using a thin nail art brush and a red nail polish, draw two vertical lines curving inward, one on each side of the nail, to make the seams of the ball.

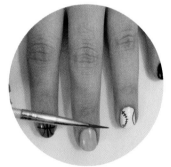 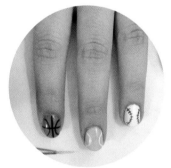 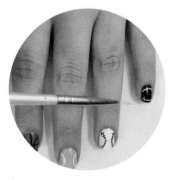

6 Using the same tool and nail polish, place short strokes along the lines to indicate the stitching.

7 For the tennis nail: Using a nail art brush and a white nail polish, draw two vertical lines curving inward, one on each side of the yellow nail.

8 For the football nail: Using a nail art brush and a white nail polish, draw two horizontal curved lines, one at the top and one at the bottom of the dark brown nail.

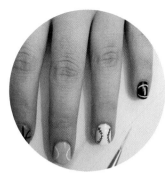

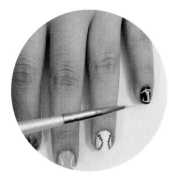

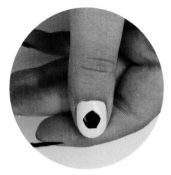

9 Using the same tool and nail polish, draw a white vertical line straight down the middle.

10 Using the same tool and nail polish, place short white strokes along the white line to indicate the stitching.

11 For the soccer nail: Using a nail art brush and a black nail polish, draw a pentagon in the center of the white nail. Fill in the pentagon with the black nail polish.

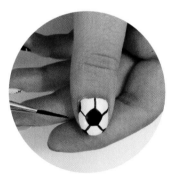

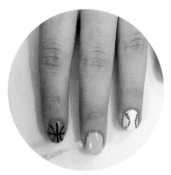

12 Using the same tool and nail polish, draw a straight black line radiating out from each point of the pentagon.

13 Finally, apply a top coat to your nails to seal in the design.

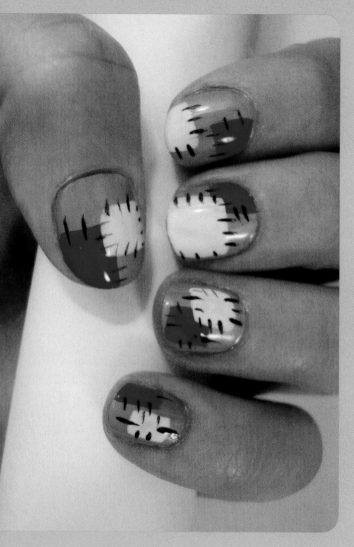

PATCHED NAILS

This cute design looks like patches sewn on your nails.

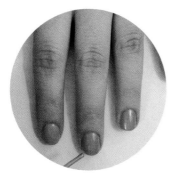 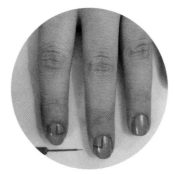 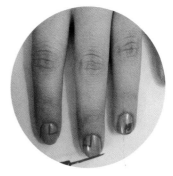

1 Start by painting your nails with a light pink nail polish.

2 Using a nail art brush and a red nail polish, draw square shapes on your nails.

3 Using the same tool and nail polish, fill in the squares with red.

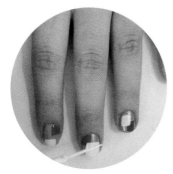 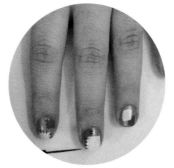 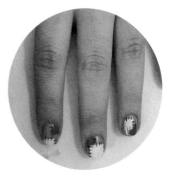

4 Using a nail art brush and a white nail polish, draw more squares on your nails and fill them in.

5 Using a thin nail art brush and a black nail polish, draw stitch lines along the edges of the squares.

6 Finally, apply a top coat to your nails to seal in the design.

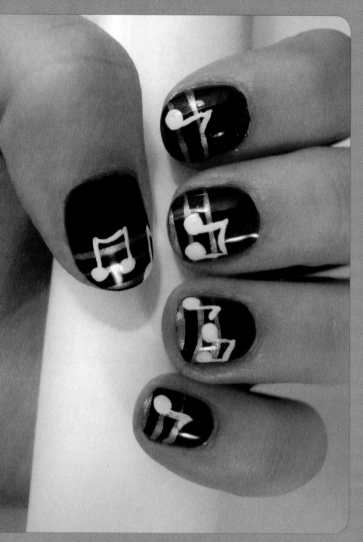

MUSIC NOTE NAILS

Simple to create, this nail art design will be music to your ears.

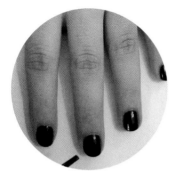

1 Start by painting your nails with a dark purple nail polish.

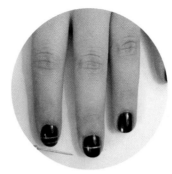

2 Using a nail art brush and a gold nail polish, create three straight horizontal lines on all of your nails.

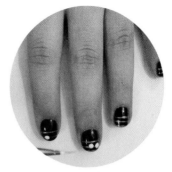

3 Using a nail art brush and a white nail polish, place dots randomly along the lines on your nails.

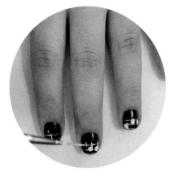

4 Using the same tool and nail polish, add a vertical line to the dot to create the music notes.

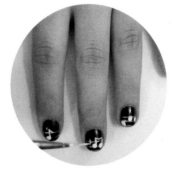

5 Using the same tool and nail polish, add a short diagonal line to the top of the note or connect two notes to create eighth notes.

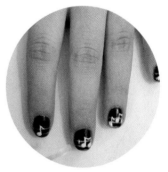

6 Finally, apply a top coat to your nails to seal in the design.

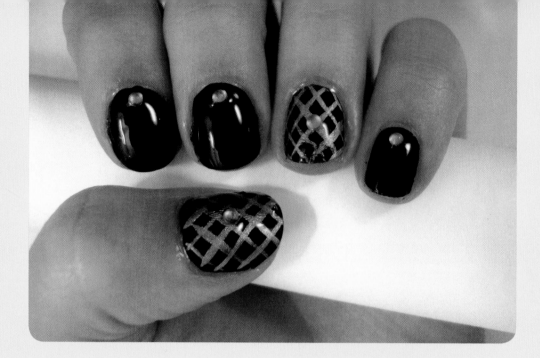

BLACK AND GOLD
JEWELED NAILS

If you're looking for a great way to dress up
your nails, this elegant design is perfect for
any event.

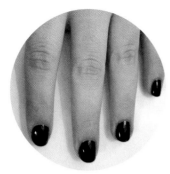

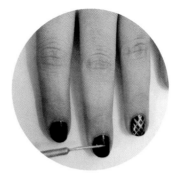

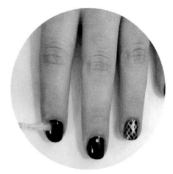

1 Start by painting your nails with a black nail polish.

2 Using a nail art brush and a gold nail polish, create a crisscross pattern on the ring finger and thumb nails.

3 Working on one nail at a time, apply a clear nail polish.

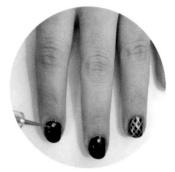

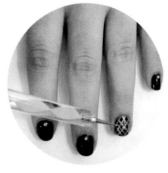

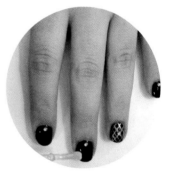

4 Carefully use a dotting tool or pair of tweezers to place a rhinestone decal in the upper middle of each nail except the ring finger and thumb nails. Be sure to do this before the clear nail polish dries, as the nail polish acts as the adhesive.

5 On the ring finger and thumb nails, carefully use a dotting tool or pair of tweezers to place the rhinestone decal at the center of the nails.

6 Finally, apply a top coat to your nails to seal in the design.

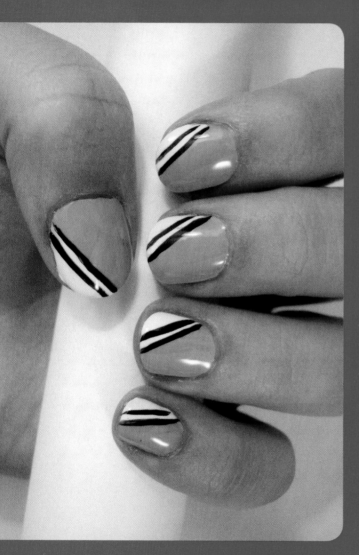

BLACK, WHITE, AND BLUE NAILS

Travel back in time to the 1950s with this classic nail art design.

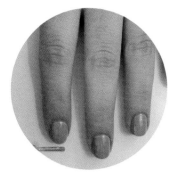

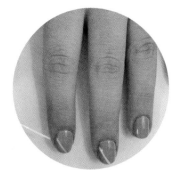

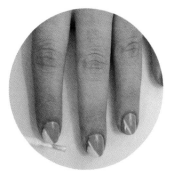

1 Start by painting your nails with a light blue nail polish.

2 Using a nail art brush and a white nail polish, draw a diagonal on the edge of the nail.

3 Using the same tool and nail polish, fill in the area with white.

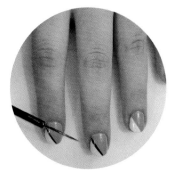

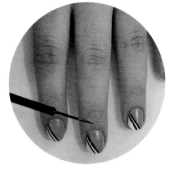

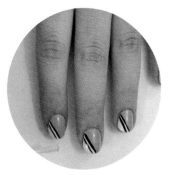

4 Using a nail art brush and a black nail polish, draw a diagonal line dividing the white and blue colors.

5 Using the same tool and nail polish, place another black diagonal line below the first black line.

6 Finally, apply a top coat to your nails to seal in the design.

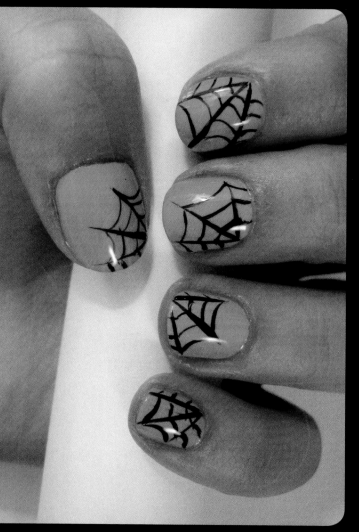

SPIDERWEB NAILS

······································

These creepy webs are the perfect addition to your favorite Halloween costume.

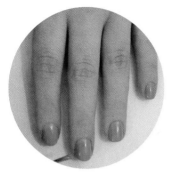

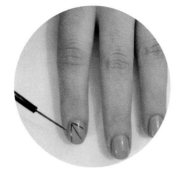

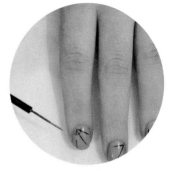

1 Start by painting your nails with a neon green nail polish.

2 Using a nail art brush and a black nail polish, draw several diagonal lines coming from the upper corner of your nail.

3 Connect the diagonal lines together with curved lines in between each line. This step will complete your spiderweb.

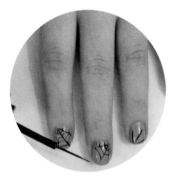

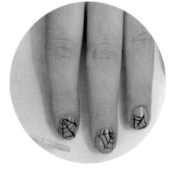

4 Continue connecting the lines together until you've reached the end of the diagonal lines.

5 Finally, apply a top coat to your nails to seal in the design.

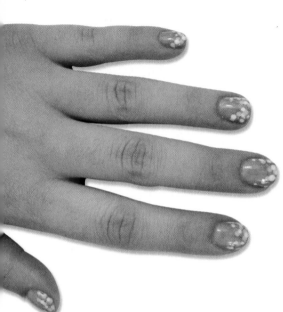

EASY DOTTED NAILS

This faded dot manicure is great for beginners: The spots are effortless, but stunning.

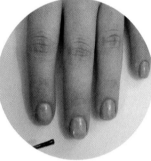

1 Start by painting your nails with a sheer pink nail polish.

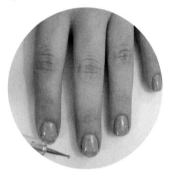

2 Using a dotting tool and a blue nail polish, place dots on your nails. Make sure to use various sizes of dots to keep things visually interesting.

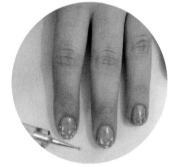

3 Repeat the previous step with pink and yellow nail polishes. Don't worry if they overlap.

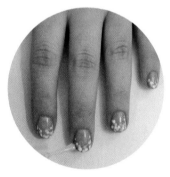

4 Finally, apply a top coat to your nails to seal in the design.

MERMAID NAILS

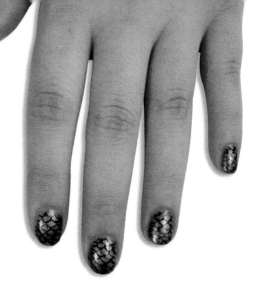

With this Atlantis-inspired design, your nails will glisten just like the sea under the sun.

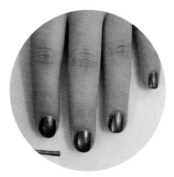

1 Start by painting your nails with a teal nail polish.

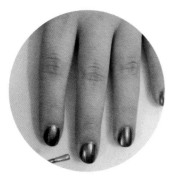

2 Lightly apply a sheer gold nail polish over the teal nail polish.

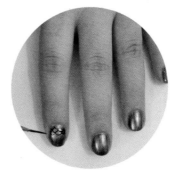

3 Using a thin nail art brush and a black nail polish, start creating curved lines on your nails in a scale design. It's okay if they overlap.

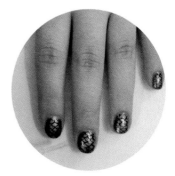

4 Finally, apply a top coat to your nails to seal in the design.

ICING TIP NAILS

Yummy icing tips are a sweet touch to your manicure.

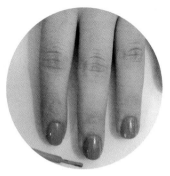

1 Start by painting your nails with a lilac nail polish.

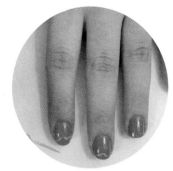

2 Using a nail art brush and a light pink nail polish, create a horizontal wavy line in the middle of your nails.

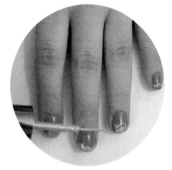

3 Fill in the bottom portion of the wave with the light pink nail polish.

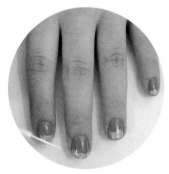

4 Using a nail art brush and a white nail polish, place short strokes on the pink area to create sprinkles.

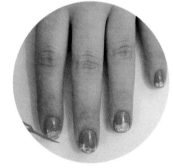

5 Repeat the previous step with a bright pink nail polish.

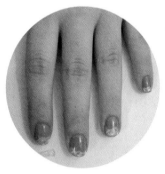

6 Finally, apply a top coat to your nails to seal in the design.

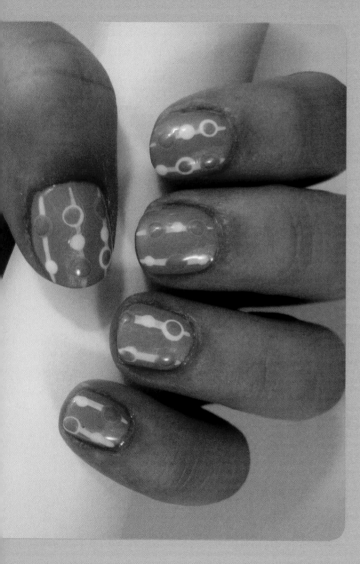

STRINGS OF DOTS NAILS

Play connect the dots with this simple but captivating design.

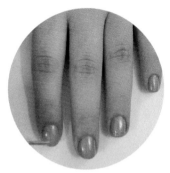

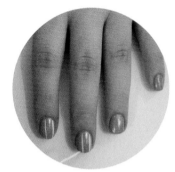

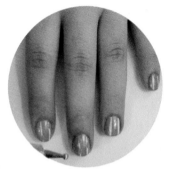

1 Start by painting your nails with a light pink nail polish.

2 Using a nail art brush and a white nail polish, draw vertical lines on your nails.

3 Using a dotting tool and a blue nail polish, place dots of various sizes on top of the lines.

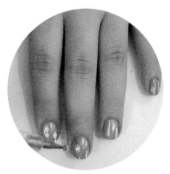

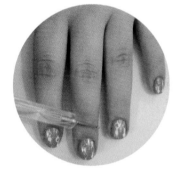

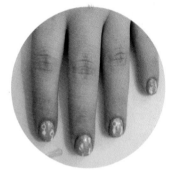

4 Repeat the previous step with a white nail polish.

5 Using the dotting tool and light pink nail polish, place smaller dots within the dots you just created.

6 Finally, apply a top coat to your nails to seal in the design.

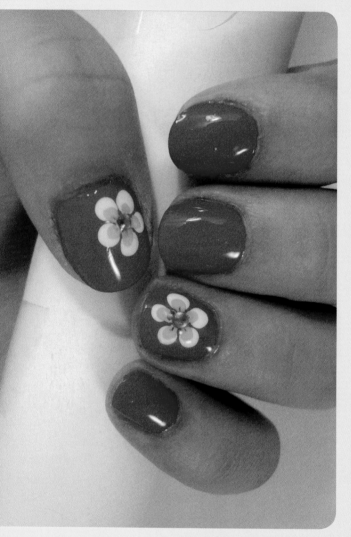

SIMPLE FLOWER NAILS

While this design may look complicated, it's actually super easy and a great starting point for beginners.

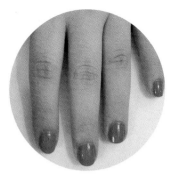

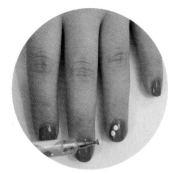

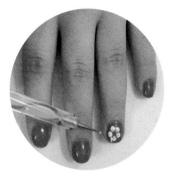

1 Start by painting your nails with a bright pink nail polish.

2 Using a dotting tool and a white nail polish, place five large dots in a circle on your thumb and ring finger nails.

3 Using the dotting tool and a yellow nail polish, place smaller dots inside the ones you just created.

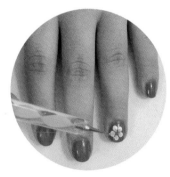

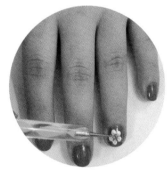

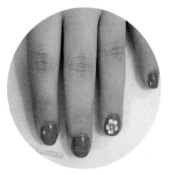

4 Before this smaller dot dries, drag the edges of each inner circle to the center with the dotting tool, so that each circle is more of a teardrop shape, and all five dots are touching.

5 Carefully place a rhinestone decal in the center of the nail with the dotting tool or a pair of tweezers.

6 Finally, apply a top coat to your nails to seal in the design.